Clinical Pharmacology and Therapeutics

Editor

KATRINA L. MEALEY

VETERINARY CLINICS OF NORTH AMERICA: SMALL ANIMAL PRACTICE

www.vetsmall.theclinics.com

September 2013 • Volume 43 • Number 5

ELSEVIER

1600 John F. Kennedy Boulevard • Suite 1800 • Philadelphia, Pennsylvania, 19103-2899
http://www.vetsmall.theclinics.com

VETERINARY CLINICS OF NORTH AMERICA: SMALL ANIMAL PRACTICE Volume 43, Number 5
September 2013 ISSN 0195-5616, ISBN-13: 978-0-323-18878-4

Editor: John Vassallo; j.vassallo@elsevier.com
Developmental Editor: Susan Showalter

Veterinary Clinics of North America: Small Animal Practice (ISSN 0195-5616) is published bimonthly by Elsevier Inc., 360 Park Avenue South, New York, NY 10010-1710. Months of issue are January, March, May, July, September, and November. Business and Editorial Offices: 1600 John F. Kennedy Blvd., Ste. 1800, Philadelphia, PA 19103-2899. Customer Service Office: 3251 Riverport Lane, Maryland Heights, MO 63043. Periodicals postage paid at New York, NY and additional mailing offices. Subscription prices are $294.00 per year (domestic individuals), $473.00 per year (domestic institutions), $143.00 per year (domestic students/residents), $390.00 per year (Canadian individuals), $580.00 per year (Canadian institutions), $433.00 per year (international individuals), $580.00 per year (international institutions), and $208.00 per year (international and Canadian students/residents). To receive student/resident rate, orders must be accompained by name of affiliated institution, date of term, and the *signature* of program/residency coordinator on institution letterhead. Orders will be billed at individual rate until proof of status is received. Foreign air speed delivery is included in all *Clinics* subscription prices. All prices are subject to change without notice. **POSTMASTER:** Send address changes to *Veterinary Clinics of North America: Small Animal Practice*, Elsevier Health Sciences Division, Subscription Customer Service, 3251 Riverport Lane, Maryland Heights, MO 63043. Customer Service (orders, claims, online, change of address): Elsevier Periodicals Customer Service, Elsevier Health Sciences Division Subscription Customer Service 3251 Riverport Lane Maryland Heights, MO 63043. Tel: 1-800-654-2452 (U.S. and Canada); 314-447-8871 (outside U.S. and Canada). Fax: 314-447-8029. E-mail: journalscustomerservice-usa@elsevier.com (for print support); journalsonlinesupport-usa@elsevier.com (for online support).

Reprints. For copies of 100 or more of articles in this publication, please contact the Commercial Reprints Department, Elsevier Inc., 360 Park Avenue South, New York, NY 10010-1710. Tel.: 212-633-3812; Fax: 212-462-1935; E-mail: reprints@elsevier.com.

Veterinary Clinics of North America: Small Animal Practice is also published in Japanese by Inter Zoo Publishing Co., Ltd., Aoyama Crystal-Bldg 5F, 3-5-12 Kitaaoyama, Minato-ku, Tokyo 107-0061, Japan.

Veterinary Clinics of North America: Small Animal Practice is covered in *Current Contents/Agriculture, Biology and Environmental Sciences, Science Citation Index, ASCA, MEDLINE/PubMed (Index Medicus), Excerpta Medica,* and *BIOSIS*.

Printed and bound by CPI Group (UK) Ltd, Croydon, CR0 4YY

Transferred to digital print 2012

Contributors

EDITOR

KATRINA L. MEALEY, DVM, PhD
Diplomate, American College of Veterinary Internal Medicine; Diplomate, American College of Veterinary Clinical Pharmacology; Individualized Medicine Program, Department of Veterinary Clinical Sciences, College of Veterinary Medicine, Washington State University, Pullman, Washington

AUTHORS

CAROLE CAMBIER, PhD
Unit of Pharmacology, Department of Functional Sciences, Faculty of Veterinary Medicine, University of Liège, Liège, Belgium

MICHAEL H. COURT, BVSc, PhD
Professor, Department of Veterinary Clinical Sciences, College of Veterinary Medicine, Washington State University, Pullman, Washington

PASCAL GUSTIN, PhD
Unit of Pharmacology, Department of Functional Sciences, Faculty of Veterinary Medicine, University of Liège, Liège, Belgium

BUTCH KUKANICH, DVM, PhD
Diplomate, American College of Veterinary Clinical Pharmacology; Associate Professor, Department of Anatomy and Physiology, Kansas State University, Manhattan, Kansas

KATRINA L. MEALEY, DVM, PhD
Diplomate, American College of Veterinary Internal Medicine; Diplomate, American College of Veterinary Clinical Pharmacology; Individualized Medicine Program, Department of Veterinary Clinical Sciences, College of Veterinary Medicine, Washington State University, Pullman, Washington

SANJA MODRIC, DVM, PhD
Office of New Animal Drug Evaluation, Center for Veterinary Medicine, Rockville, Maryland

KAREN R. MUÑANA, DVM, MS
Diplomate, American College of Veterinary Internal Medicine (Neurology); Department of Clinical Sciences, College of Veterinary Medicine, North Carolina State University, Raleigh, North Carolina

MARK G. PAPICH, DVM, MS
Diplomate, American College of Veterinary Clinical Pharmacology; Professor of Clinical Pharmacology, College of Veterinary Medicine, North Carolina State University, Raleigh, North Carolina

LAUREN A. TREPANIER, DVM, PhD
Diplomate, American College of Veterinary Internal Medicine; Diplomate, American College of Veterinary Clinical Pharmacology; Professor of Internal Medicine, Department of Medical Sciences, School of Veterinary Medicine, University of Wisconsin-Madison, Madison, Wisconsin

JEAN-MICHEL VANDEWEERD, PhD
Integrated Veterinary Research Unit (IVRU), Namur Research Institute for Life Sciences (NARILIS), Department of Veterinary Medicine, University of Namur, Namur, Belgium

KATRINA R. VIVIANO, DVM, PhD
Diplomate, American College of Veterinary Internal Medicine; Diplomate, American College of Veterinary Clinical Pharmacology; Department of Medical Sciences, School of Veterinary Medicine, University of Wisconsin, Madison, Wisconsin

Contents

these differences are poorly understood. This article evaluates published evidence for altered drug effects in cats, focusing on pharmacokinetic differences between cats, dogs, and humans, and the molecular mechanisms underlying these differences. More work is needed to better understand drug metabolism and disposition differences in cats, thereby enabling more rational prescribing of existing medications, and the development of safer drugs for this species.

Idiosyncratic drug toxicity reactions are, by definition, uncommon, but can lead to serious or even fatal organ toxicity. The liver, skin, and peripheral blood cells/bone marrow are common targets. Most of these reactions are the result of reactive metabolites, which may cause local cell or organelle damage, or may be amplified by a systemic immune response. Individual risk may depend on differences in drug biotransformation, levels of oxidative stress, or antigen presentation.

For many drugs used in veterinary practice, plasma and tissue concentrations are highly dependent on the activity of drug transporters. This article describes how functional changes in drug transporters, whether mediated by genetic variability or drug-drug interactions, affect drug disposition and, ultimately, drug safety and efficacy in veterinary patients. A greater understanding of species, breed, and individual (genetic) differences in drug transporter function, as well as drug-drug interactions involving drug transporters, will result in improved strategies for drug design and will enable veterinarians to incorporate individualized medicine in their practices.

Veterinarians are quick to attribute an unsuccessful antimicrobial treatment to a failure of the culture and susceptibility test. There are many reasons why antimicrobial treatment fails. When evaluating a patient that has failed to respond to therapy, one must consider any of the many factors that contribute to antibiotic failure.

There are few veterinary clinical studies to support a recommended use and dose for treating resistant bacterial infections in small animals. Resistance against many common antibiotics is possible and a susceptibility test is advised. Infections caused by *Pseudomonas aeruginosa* presents a special problem. *Staphylococcus* isolated from small animals is most likely to be *Staphylococcus pseudintermedius*. The most important resistance mechanism for *Staphylococcus* is methicillin resistance. The only antimicrobials to which some gram-negative bacilli are sensitive may be extended-spectrum cephalosporins, carbapenems (penems), selected penicillin derivatives, amikacin, or tobramycin. A susceptibility test is needed to identify the appropriate drug for these infections.

This article evaluates the current literature on oral analgesics and analgesic adjuncts in dogs and cats. An overview of how dosing recommendations are made covering controlled clinical trials, experimental study design, and pharmacokinetic studies is included. The weight of evidence for each drug is reviewed and compared with the gold standard, controlled clinical trials. Other evidence such as experimental studies, extrapolation of pharmacokinetic studies, and case reports/series is also considered. It important to know from what data dosing recommendations are derived and how much evidence supports the use of oral analgesics and analgesic adjuncts in dogs and cats.

Seizures are the most common neurologic condition encountered in small animal practice and arise from an imbalance of excitatory and inhibitory mechanisms in the brain. Epilepsy refers to recurrent seizures of any cause. Successful management of epilepsy requires knowledge of the pharmacologic properties of available antiepileptic medications, regular patient evaluations to assess response to therapy and monitor for adverse effects, and thorough client education to ensure that goals and expectations of therapy are understood. Recommendations for emergency care of seizures at home should be provided for patients with seizures that are not controlled with maintenance antiepileptic therapy.

Treatment of immune-mediated disease in dogs and cats continues to evolve as new therapies are introduced or adapted from human medicine. Glucocorticoids remain the first-line therapy for many of the immune-mediated or inflammatory diseases of cats and dogs. The focus of this article is to provide an update on some of the common immunosuppressive therapies used in small animal veterinary medicine. The goals of therapy are to induce disease remission through the inhibition of inflammation and the modulation of lymphocyte function.

Nutraceuticals, or nutritional supplements, have been promoted for the ancillary treatment of liver disease in dogs. However, minimal information is available in the scientific literature about commonly used nutraceuticals, such as *S*-adenosylmethionine, silymarin, and vitamin E. No strong clinical evidence exists regarding the efficacy of these compounds as hepatoprotectants in canine liver disease. Until this evidence exists, individual veterinarians must assume responsibility for their decision to use nutritional supplements in their canine patients with liver disease.

VETERINARY CLINICS OF NORTH AMERICA: SMALL ANIMAL PRACTICE

RELATED INTEREST

Veterinary Clinics of North America: Equine Practice
April 2013, Volume 29, Number 1
Topics in Equine Anesthesia
Stuart C. Clark-Price, DVM, MS, *Editor*

THE CLINICS ARE NOW AVAILABLE ONLINE!
Access your subscription at:
www.theclinics.com

Preface

Clinical Pharmacology and Therapeutics

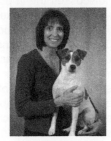

Katrina L. Mealey, DVM, PhD
Editor

Seven years ago, Dr Dawn Merton Boothe served as guest editor of the last Clinical Pharmacology issue of the *Veterinary Clinics of North America: Small Animal Practice* (September 2006). Each of the topics addressed in that issue are still relevant today, and the current issue provides updates on many of these important topics. The authors of the articles in this issue are nationally and internationally recognized experts in their respective fields and their articles are packed with valuable information for veterinary students, practicing veterinarians, and clinical pharmacologists. The rationale for selecting the topics included in this issue is discussed below.

Recent events involving multiple human and veterinary patients receiving either contaminated or inaccurately compounded drugs have resulted in numerous deaths, national media coverage, and, in my opinion, long overdue legislative attention focused on compounded drug products. Because of the severity of these errors by compounding pharmacies, it is likely that the FDA's role in regulating compounding pharmacies will change over the next several years. In the meantime, it seemed prudent to include information about use of approved and unapproved drugs for veterinary practitioners. Sanja Modric, DVM, PhD, of the FDA Center for Veterinary Medicine, provides important information for veterinarians to consider when deciding between an FDA-approved drug that has been tested for safety, efficacy, and quality versus an untested compounded product.

Since the last Clinical Pharmacology issue, awareness of the extent to which pharmacogenetics influences drug disposition has increased, not only in human medicine but in veterinary medicine as well. This is exemplified by the launch of the first Individualized Veterinary Medicine program at Washington State University College of Veterinary Medicine. This program is similar to the Personalized Medicine programs

Vet Clin Small Anim 43 (2013) xi–xiii
http://dx.doi.org/10.1016/j.cvsm.2013.05.004
0195-5616/13/$ – see front matter © 2013 Published by Elsevier Inc.

vetsmall.theclinics.com

offered by many medical schools. This cluster of articles begins with an introductory article (applying pharmacokinetics to clinical veterinary practice) that reacquaints the reader with terminology first introduced in veterinary pharmacology courses. Lauren Trepanier, DVM, PhD, provides clinically relevant and easy-to-understand examples of how to adjust drug doses in response to changes in any of the common pharmacokinetic parameters (whether those changes are mediated by disease states, genetic differences, or drug interactions). Michael Court, BVSc, PhD, discusses the importance of cytochrome P450 enzymes in the context of pharmacogenetics and the likelihood that discoveries in the near future may allow prediction (and therefore, prevention) of some adverse drug reactions in canine patients. Dr Court also examines differences in feline drug disposition as compared to that of dogs and humans. Although many drugs are eliminated more slowly in cats than in dogs or humans, some are actually eliminated faster. Dr Court's findings suggest that while metabolic conjugation reactions are slower in cats, some oxidation reactions may be more rapid in cats. The pharmacogenetic (molecular) mechanisms for some of these differences are described. Updates on the role of pharmacogenetics in idiosyncratic adverse drug reactions and the role of drug transporter pharmacogenetics are also included. The article on drug transporters provides information on MDR1 genetic testing for dogs (MDR1 genotyping is used to prevent life-threatening adverse drug reactions in dogs).

Because of the continued emergence of multidrug-resistant bacterial pathogens, veterinarians face increasing scrutiny in our use of antimicrobial drugs in all veterinary patients, even dogs and cats. A thorough understanding of susceptibility testing and how to interpret (Minimal Inhibitory Concentration MIC) data is more important now than ever. Mark Papich, DVM, MS, has provided 2 articles with up-to-date information on new veterinary-specific MIC data, newer concepts in susceptibility testing, and strategies for treating resistant bacterial infections.

Three therapeutic areas that seemed in need of an update are also included as separate articles. Although newer NSAIDs have enabled veterinarians to provide outpatients with improved pain control, NSAIDs are not the optimal choice for analgesia in all patients. An increasing number of human drugs are being used in an extralabel manner to treat pain in canine and feline patients. In some instances, very little evidence exists to support the use of these drugs in dogs and cats. Butch KuKanich, DVM, PhD, provides a clinically relevant, evidence-based review of outpatient analgesics that may be alternatives or adjuncts to NSAIDs. Since the last issue was published, more than 20 new studies involving seizure management in dogs or cats have been published. Many of these drugs are human drug products used in an extralabel manner so these studies provide critical information about the safety and efficacy of these drugs in dogs and cats with seizure disorders. Karen Muñana, DVM, MS, has provided a clinically relevant, evidence-based assessment of novel antiepileptic drug therapy in dogs and cats. Similarly, Katrina Viviano, DVM, PhD, has provided an update on immunosuppressive therapies for dogs and cats. Novel information includes an evidence-based assessment of the newer "topical" corticosteroids approved for human respiratory and gastrointestinal inflammatory diseases, tacrolimus, the accumulated data on cyclosporine, and a few other human immunosuppressive therapies.

Because of the popularity of using nutritional supplements as "hepatoprotectants," a review of the literature using an evidence-based approach seemed overdue. Jean-Michel Vandeweerd, DMV, MSc, PhD, recently published a systematic review of the efficacy of so-called nutraceuticals for treating osteoarthritis. He was asked to provide a similar review for nutritional supplements promoted for use as hepatoprotectants in dogs.

Each of the authors is extremely busy with numerous demands placed on their time and I am grateful that they agreed to author articles in this issue.

Katrina L. Mealey, DVM, PhD
Department of Veterinary Clinical Sciences
Individualized Medicine Program
College of Veterinary Medicine
Washington State University
Pullman, WA 99164-6610, USA

E-mail address:
kmealey@vetmed.wsu.edu

Regulatory Framework for the Availability and Use of Animal Drugs in the United States

Sanja Modric, DVM, PhD

KEYWORDS

- Drug approval process • Approved versus unapproved drugs • Regulatory • Safety

KEY POINTS

- Use by veterinarians of animal drugs approved by the Food and Drug Administration (FDA) is the only way to be assured of product safety and efficacy, truthful and complete labeling, and appropriate manufacturing standards.
- Statements made on product labels or Web sites such as "made in an FDA-registered facility" or "registered and listed with the FDA" does not mean that product is an FDA-approved drug.
- FDA-approved drugs can be identified by searching the online database Animal Drugs @ FDA or by identifying the 6-digit NADA or ANADA number on the product label.

INTRODUCTION

Given the relatively limited number of approved animal drugs available to veterinarians, practitioners often rely on the use of various types and sources of drugs to treat their patients. Some of these products may be unapproved for human and/or animal use, they may be unsafe or have no discernible clinical effect, or they may lack a solid pharmacologic basis for their use. Only when buying animal drugs approved by the US Food and Drug Administration (FDA) are practitioners assured of the product safety, effectiveness, and manufacturing to the strict standards for quality, purity, and potency. However, even when using approved veterinary products, companion animal veterinarians may not always be aware of the specific condition(s) of use for which

Disclosures: The author has nothing to disclose.
This article represents a compilation of information available in a variety of documents available on the CVM Web site (http://www.fda.gov/AnimalVeterinary/default.htm) and the original material by the author. The reader is encouraged to visit the Web site for more detailed information on each of the topics covered in this article.
Office of New Animal Drug Evaluation, Center for Veterinary Medicine, 7500 Standish Place, Rockville, MD 20855, USA
E-mail address: sanja.modric@fda.hhs.gov

a drug is approved, such as the indication(s), dose and dosing regimen, target species, and route of administration. Because of these conditions of use, a product approved, for example, for the treatment of skin infections associated with specific susceptible bacteria indicated on the label may not be effective for treating other types of infections, or the dose for other infections may not be adequate. In addition, if a higher dose or a different dosing regimen is used than is stated on the approved product label, there is an increased risk of toxicity, as the safety has not been evaluated at those higher doses and/or more frequent dosing regimens.

It may be difficult for practitioners to recognize the differences between approved and unapproved drugs (or uses), and understand and appreciate potential risks associated with the use of unapproved or approved products used outside of the approved label conditions. The risks may range from mild adverse reactions or poor efficacy response to life-threatening toxicity or complete lack of effectiveness, both of which may ultimately result in the patient's harm. Therefore, it is critical for practitioners in modern veterinary practice to not only use and understand drug labels and how they may affect their patients, but also to check them periodically for updates of important safety information.

The goal of this introductory article is to help practitioners understand the basis for the approval of new animal drugs, the terminology and specific meaning of terms related to the approval, and the marketing and use of veterinary drugs in companion animal practice.

The FDA Center for Veterinary Medicine (CVM) regulates the manufacture and distribution of drugs and food additives that will be given to animals. Animal drugs are regulated under The Federal Food, Drug, and Cosmetic Act (FFDCA; the Act), which provides the statutory provisions governing the regulation of veterinary products. The Act defines the term *drugs*, in part, as "articles intended for use in the diagnosis, cure, mitigation, treatment, or prevention of disease in man or other animals" and "articles (other than food) intended to affect the structure or any function of the body of man or other animals." Under the Act, a *new animal drug* is considered to be unsafe unless there is an approved New Animal Drug Application (NADA) or Abbreviated New Animal Drug Application (ANADA) under section 512 of the FFDCA, a conditional approval under section 571, or an index listing under section 572.

REGULATORY PATHWAYS FOR APPROVAL OF NEW ANIMAL DRUGS

There are several different legal pathways for the approval of animal drugs. Drugs can be approved by submitting a NADA and obtaining a new animal drug approval, or by submitting an ANADA and obtaining a generic animal drug approval. The FDA's approval means the drug is safe and effective when it is used according to the label; its strength, quality, and purity are consistent from batch to batch; and its labeling is truthful and complete.

Before a new animal drug is approved, the sponsor must establish, among other things, that the drug is safe and effective for the intended use, that its manufacturing complies with quality requirements, and that the labeling is truthful and complete. There are 6 data elements (commonly referred to as technical sections) that must be completed for a new companion animal drug approval: Effectiveness; Target Animal Safety (TAS); Chemistry, Manufacturing, and Controls (CMC); Environmental Safety; All Other Information; and Labeling. Approved new animal drugs can be categorized as either brand name or generic.

- A *brand-name (pioneer) new animal drug* is an original FDA-approved new animal drug marketed under a proprietary, trademark-protected name. The new animal drug approval process includes a detailed and comprehensive review of all the submitted data as described above (recently reviewed by Smith and Modric, 2013[1]). The process is very similar for drugs intended for food-producing and companion animals, with the exception that a human food safety evaluation is not required for drugs intended for use in companion animals. After an approved brand-name animal drug has been on the market for a specific number of years, another drug sponsor can start the approval process for a generic copy by submitting an ANADA.

- A *generic new animal drug* is a copy of an approved new animal drug that has been previously approved and shown to be safe and effective when used in accordance with its labeling. For the approval of a generic animal drug, the information in the ANADA must show that the active ingredients of a generic animal drug are the same as those of the approved product and that it is bioequivalent to the approved animal drug product. The finished product must also be the same strength and dosage form, with the same route of administration, as the approved product. The application is "abbreviated" because generic copies of brand-name animal drugs go through a shortened drug approval process, allowing sponsors to fulfill TAS and effectiveness requirements through the demonstration of product bioequivalence (established in 1988 by the Generic Animal Drug and Patent Term Restoration Act). Similar to the brand-name drug approval, the information in the ANADA must also show that the generic copy is consistently made from batch to batch and that the labeling for the generic copy must match the labeling for the approved brand-name animal drug, except for a few allowable differences (eg, a different trade name).

Once approved, both brand-name and generic animal drugs can have subsequent supplemental approvals that legally extend an approved product's conditions of use. Supplemental new animal drug applications allow companies to make changes to an approved product while relying on the existing approval for some of the application requirements. Depending on the type of changes proposed in supplemental applications, new effectiveness and TAS data may or may not be required. Minor changes (such as a change in container style, shape, size or components; a minor change in the manufacturing processes; the addition of an alternative manufacturer) do not require additional safety and/or effectiveness information. By contrast, major changes (such as a change in dose or treatment regimen, the addition of a new species, or the addition of a new claim) can affect the safety and/or effectiveness of the new animal drug, and thus need to be evaluated before supplemental approval and indication on the new label. This new labeling information may be of great importance to practitioners when selecting drug treatment for their patients because of new effectiveness and/or safety information.

The FDA is responsible for determining the marketing status of animal drug products based on the ability to provide adequate directions for safe and effective use of the product by a lay person:

- *Prescription* (Rx) products can be dispensed only by or upon the lawful written order of a licensed veterinarian.
- *Over-the-counter* (OTC) drugs have labels written so that the layman can use a drug safely and for the purposes for which it is intended (adequate directions for use).
- *Veterinary Feed Directive* (VFD) is a written statement issued by a licensed veterinarian to authorize the client to obtain and use the VFD drug in or on animal feed in accordance with the directions for use approved by the FDA.

The same drug substance can be approved and marketed in several different dosage forms, intended for use by different routes of administration and in different species of animals. Therefore, the same drug substance may be distributed OTC for one use or application and by prescription use only for another use or application. In addition, the marketing status may change after the initial approval, thus encouraging practitioners to regularly check drug labeling.

MINOR USE AND MINOR SPECIES CONSIDERATIONS

Animal drugs intended to be used in minor species and/or for minor uses have additional unique aspects for approval and marketing. Many of these drugs came into being through passage of The Minor Use and Minor Species (MUMS) Animal Health Act of 2004. This law is intended to encourage pharmaceutical firms to make more medications legally available to veterinarians and animal owners, to treat minor animal species and uncommon diseases in the major animal species. The legal definition of minor species in the United States includes all species other than humans and the major species (ie, cattle, horses, swine, chickens, turkeys, dogs, and cats). "Minor use" (in major species) is defined as diseases that occur infrequently or in limited geographic areas and in only a small number of animals annually. The "small number" for each of the major species is defined by regulation.

A common challenge for drug approvals in minor species is the animal diversity (eg, zoo animals, ornamental fish, parrots, ferrets, guinea pigs) and the limited number of animals that can be used in effectiveness and safety testing. In addition, there is a vast difference in animal care and management, diseases, and inherent sensitivity to or toxicity of pharmaceutical products. Many of these same limitations apply to the uncommon diseases or conditions in the major species.

The MUMS Act provides several innovative ways to encourage development and approval/marketing of drugs used either in minor species or to treat uncommon diseases in major species. Although many drugs may be available to veterinarians under the extralabel drug use (ELDU) provisions, they are not approved for these particular uses. Effectiveness and safety information for the ELDU is not available for the specific unique use, but would become available through the MUMS approval process. Also, many minor species are most effectively treated using medicated feeds, which are not permitted to be used outside their labeling.

Minor use/minor species animal drugs are eligible to complete a *Conditional New Animal Drug Application* (CNADA), and can obtain a conditional approval. This process has the same approval requirements as the NADA process with the exception of effectiveness. For a new animal drug application, the effectiveness has to be demonstrated before drug approval through independent substantiation in adequate and well-controlled studies (Code of Federal Regulations, 21 CFR 514.117) and by providing valid inferences to the target population (inferential value). For a conditional approval, however, drugs have to demonstrate a reasonable expectation of effectiveness. Following conditional approval, drugs can be legally marketed for up to 5 years, through annual renewals, while collecting the remaining required effectiveness data to fulfill all NADA requirements.

Another process unique to MUMS drugs, Designation, is an incentive program that encourages development of drugs for minor species or rare diseases. Sponsors of "designated" new animal drugs are eligible to apply for grants to fund safety and effectiveness studies, and also receive 7 years of exclusive marketing rights for the designated use of their new animal drug beginning on the date of approval or conditional approval.

Yet another unique and innovative approach that the MUMS Act provides is legal marketing of some unapproved new animal drugs for non–food-producing minor species, based largely on a scientific evaluation of effectiveness and safety by an outside expert panel. Drugs in this category may be added to the *Index of Legally Marketed Unapproved New Animal Drugs for Minor Species* (the Index). Indexed drugs, although not approved, provide specific information for practitioners and users regarding the dose, indications, and safe use of such products. This process is easier and less costly for sponsors interested in achieving legal marketing status for products for minor species (eg, zoo animals, ornamental fish, reptiles, caged birds), for which the approval process would likely be cost-prohibitive and/or impractical owing to the scarcity and inherent value of the animals.

EXTRALABEL DRUG USE

ELDU refers to the use of an approved drug in a manner that is not in accordance with the approved label indications. Until the passing of the Animal Medicinal Drug Use Clarification Act of 1994 (AMDUCA), the ELDU of new animal drugs was considered illegal, and the FDA exercised enforcement discretion under certain circumstances. AMDUCA amended the FFDCA to allow for ELDU by or on the order of a licensed veterinarian within the context of a valid veterinarian-client-patient relationship under certain conditions.

ELDU is common in companion animal practice because the number of available approved animal drugs is relatively small, and those that are approved are approved for specific conditions of use. Drugs can be used in an extralabel manner if there is no animal drug approved for the intended use; an animal drug is approved but in a different dosage form or concentration; or the approved drug has been found to be clinically ineffective when used as labeled. However, in any case, the product used in an extralabel manner has to be an FDA-approved (human or veterinary) drug.

Veterinary involvement is required for ELDU because there is no direct evidence of the safety and effectiveness of the drug for the unapproved indication, dose, species, and so forth. When a drug is used by or under the supervision of a veterinarian, it decreases potential risks of toxicity and/or lack of effectiveness associated with ELDU. Therefore, a veterinarian is needed to not only diagnose a disease and make the optimal therapeutic selection for a specific individual patient, but also to continue monitoring the animal's progress and make necessary adjustments. Veterinary involvement is particularly critical for animals for which there is a dearth of approved products and a general lack of understanding as to how such products may be used safely and effectively (eg, zoo animals, exotic pets).

UNAPPROVED VERSUS APPROVED DRUGS

Unapproved animal drugs include traditional drugs used in veterinary practice (some injectable vitamins, medicated shampoos, intravenous glucose solution, antidotes, and so forth), animal supplements, homeopathic remedies, other complementary/alternative medicine products, and products compounded from bulk. The problems with using unapproved products are that: (1) they are not reviewed by the FDA and may not meet the FDA's strict standards for safety and effectiveness; (2) they may not be labeled or advertised appropriately or truthfully; and (3) manufacture of these products may not maintain the drug's quality, purity, and consistency. In addition, any safety, effectiveness, and/or manufacturing problems with these drugs are difficult to identify because there are no reporting requirements of adverse drug events for unapproved animal drugs. By contrast, as part of the FDA's continued monitoring of safety and effectiveness, drug companies are legally required to report to the FDA all adverse drug events that occur after the drug is approved. The required reporting of adverse drug events allows the FDA to more easily identify problems and provide additional labeling language or to take other safety measures (as deemed necessary) after a drug is approved and used in a large number of patients. Such safety monitoring throughout the life cycle of a drug is not available for drugs that are not approved by the FDA.

The goal of the FDA-approval process is to protect animals and humans from unsafe, ineffective, and/or substandard products by providing safe and effective approved products. Drug companies that make and sell unapproved animal drugs potentially put the health of animals (and perhaps people) at risk. Veterinarians can decide whether the risks of using such products outweigh the expected benefits, but the risk-to-benefit evaluation should be based on the knowledge and understanding of the drug being used as well as its source. Practitioners selecting an FDA-approved drug can have confidence that the drug will have the effect it purports to have on the labeling. Using FDA-approved drugs decreases the health risks associated with unapproved drug use.

There are multiple ways practitioners can tell whether the product they are using is approved or not:

- All FDA-approved animal drugs have a 6-digit NADA or ANADA number on the label. The statement "Approved by FDA" is usually on the drug label.
- Most prescription and over-the counter FDA-approved animal drugs are listed in a searchable online database, Animal Drugs @ FDA. The database allows one to search using several parameters, including proprietary name (trade name), active ingredient, application (NADA or ANADA) number, dosage form, species, and indications.
- Most FDA-approved animal drugs are also included in the "Green Book," another database available on the CVM Web site, which is updated monthly.

There are several common misconceptions among veterinarians about the approval status of animal drugs available in veterinary practice. For example, the presence of a National Drug Code (NDC) number on an animal drug label does not mean that the drug is approved by the FDA. Similarly, the statement "Caution: Federal law restricts this drug to use by or on the order of a licensed veterinarian" does not mean that it is an FDA-approved drug. Furthermore, manufacturers of unapproved drugs may put other statements on their label that may suggest that their products are approved, such as: "Registered and listed with the FDA"; "Made in an FDA-registered facility"; "Made in an FDA-inspected facility"; "Made in an FDA-approved facility." None of these statements mean that the product is approved by the FDA, but because they contain the abbreviation FDA, they are misleading and are commonly interpreted as "FDA approved."

Finally, when choosing pharmacologic treatment for their patients, practitioners should also be aware of long-term effects of using unapproved animal drugs on veterinary practice and animal health. Drug companies that make and sell these unapproved animal drugs compete against drug companies that spend time and financial resources on seeking approval from the FDA. If the market is full of unapproved drugs, drug companies may be less willing to obtain approval for animal drugs. Ultimately, this may result in a decreased availability of safe and effective new animal drugs in the United States.

POSTAPPROVAL MONITORING AND REPORTING OF ADVERSE DRUG EXPERIENCE

Monitoring of veterinary drugs to assure their continued safety and effectiveness is one of the critical roles of the CVM. Evaluation of drug safety and efficacy continues throughout a drug's life cycle through postapproval adverse drug experience (ADE) reporting to the FDA, which is mandatory for sponsors marketing approved animal drugs. The primary purpose of the CVM ADE database is to provide an early warning or signaling system to the CVM for adverse effects not detected during premarket testing of FDA-approved animal drugs.

Adverse drug experience includes, but is not limited to: (1) An adverse event occurring in animals in the course of the use of an animal drug product by a veterinarian or by a livestock producer or other animal owner or caretaker; (2) Failure of a new animal drug to produce its expected pharmacological or clinical effect (lack of expected effectiveness); and (3) An adverse event occurring in humans from exposure during manufacture, testing, handling, or use of a new animal drug. (21 CFR 514.3)

Inclusion of a good medical history, all concomitant medications the animal is on, any recent surgical procedures, and as many clinical findings as possible helps the FDA evaluate the reported ADE to determine how likely it is to be drug related. Clinical findings including veterinary examination, clinical chemistries, complete blood counts, urinalysis, fecal examinations, radiographic results, and hemodynamic data such as blood pressure, any other pressure measurements in or around the heart, and neurologic assessments are all helpful in the assessment of each individual report.

Data on adverse events do have limitations because of various possible confounding factors that may play a role in reported toxicity or ineffectiveness. Factors such as concomitant medications, preexisting medical conditions, environmental conditions, and unapproved use of FDA-approved drugs (eg, different dose, dosage regimen, and/or species) need to be considered when determining whether the adverse effect may be correlated with the drug treatment. Because ADEs are reported from animal populations of uncertain size, it is not possible to reliably estimate incidence rates. Although drug companies report the quantity of drugs marketed each year, it is not possible to determine the actual number of animals treated (because most small animal drugs are administered on an mg/kg basis), which would provide a better estimate of drug use.

Despite its limitations, the monitoring and evaluation of ADE reports is critical for ensuring adequate drug performance and preventing adverse health effects in animals. The CVM publishes a cumulative summary of ADE reports with a listing of clinical signs reported for each active ingredient in the database. Clinical signs are listed in order from most frequently observed to least frequently observed, by species and route of administration. This information can be very useful for clinicians, especially regarding new drugs, because the signs are reported much more quickly than any label changes can be made. By regularly checking the ADE report summaries veterinarians can be alerted early about potential safety concerns, and can decide to reconsider their drug selection or monitor their patients more closely. Although the ADE reporting cannot be used to estimate incidence rates or drug risk (because there is no accurate way to determine how many animals were given the drug), the frequency of reported signs will alert practitioners to pay particular attention to specific types of adverse events.

The CVM encourages veterinarians and animal owners to be vigilant and active participants in reporting adverse events and suspected product failures to help identify potential problems as early as possible. The CVM recommends that veterinarians contact the drug company to report an ADE for their product and to ask to speak to a technical services veterinarian. Telephone numbers of drug companies can usually be obtained from product labeling. The technical services veterinarian should ask a series of questions about the event, complete the FDA 1932 form, and forward the report to the CVM. If the drug is not approved by the FDA, or if it is approved but the clinician does not want to contact the manufacturer, the ADE can be reported directly to the FDA on Form 1932a.

In summary, knowledge gained from ADE data is an important surveillance tool for continuous monitoring of drug safety and for veterinarians to learn about safety concerns that may not have been observed (or noticeable) during the drug approval process. However, the only way to maximize the ADE reporting value is through a concerted effort and commitment from practitioners, animal owners, manufacturers, and regulators to collect and report good-quality data that can be further analyzed and assessed for potential safety risks.

SUMMARY

Small animal practitioners have a variety of pharmacologic options in selecting the optimal treatment for their patients. However, the level of confidence in selecting the best treatment depends on the quality of information available to the practitioner on the safe and effective use of drugs. Understanding the differences between FDA-approved versus unapproved drugs and approved versus unapproved uses helps practitioners in making the right treatment decisions. Only when buying FDA-approved animal drugs are clinicians assured of the product safety, effectiveness, and manufacturing to the strict standards for quality, purity, and potency, and that the labeling is truthful and complete. It is critical for practitioners in modern veterinary practice to not only use drug labels and understand how they may affect their patients, but also to check them periodically for updates on important safety information.

Finally, the CVM Web site, http://www.fda.gov/AnimalVeterinary/default.htm, contains a wealth of information for veterinarians, consumers, and other parties interested in animal and veterinary topics. The free e-mail alert service allows subscribers to receive important CVM news and information as it becomes available. In addition, the CVM has a Twitter account, http://www.twitter.com/FDAanimalhealth, which provides another way to receive up-to-date information regarding veterinary drugs and medicine. Regular CVM updates allow veterinarians to remain current on new approvals for animal drugs, updated drug safety and health information, development of new drugs, current science and research at the CVM, and many other topics relevant to veterinary practice.

REFERENCE

1. Smith ER, Modric S. Regulatory Considerations for the Approval of Analgesic Drugs for Cattle in the United States. In: Coetzee editor. Veterinary Clinics of North America: Food Animal Practice 2013, 29(1). p. 1–10.

Applying Pharmacokinetics to Veterinary Clinical Practice

Lauren A. Trepanier, DVM, PhD

KEYWORDS

- Bioavailability • Drug dose adjustment • Therapeutic drug monitoring
- Drug biotransformation

KEY POINTS

- Bioavailability can be used to extrapolate dosages between administration routes.
- C_{max}:MIC and AUC:MIC ratios can guide treatment with aminoglycosides and fluoroquinolones, respectively.
- Steady-state plasma concentrations for any drug are reached in 5 elimination half-lives. These concentrations may or may not be in the therapeutic range depending on the dosage.
- The time for drug washout is also equal to 5 elimination half-lives, but elimination half-lives for any active metabolites should also be considered.
- Drug dosage adjustments in human patients with renal failure are based on creatinine clearance. Because of insufficient data in dogs and cats, human recommendations can be used a rough guide until more data are available.

INTRODUCTION

Pharmacokinetics can be thought of as everything that the body does to the drug after administration and includes absorption, distribution, metabolism, and excretion. Pharmacokinetic data are available on most drugs approved for veterinary use and are often available (in dogs) for drugs developed for human patients. Parameters such as bioavailability, C_{max}, volume of distribution, clearance, and elimination half-life may seem abstract but can be directly applied in the clinic setting to tailor drug therapy and clinical monitoring for individual patients.

Bioavailability

Bioavailability is the percentage of administered drug that appears in the bloodstream after dosing.

Disclosures: The author has nothing to disclose.
School of Veterinary Medicine, Department of Medical Sciences, University of Wisconsin-Madison, 2015 Linden Drive, Madison, WI 53706-1102, USA
E-mail address: latrepanier@svm.vetmed.wisc.edu

Bioavailability after intravenous (IV) dosing is, by definition, 100%, and other routes are often compared with the IV route. Oral bioavailability is affected by drug size, lipophilicity, charge, and binding to dietary constituents (**Table 1**). For example, ciprofloxacin has poor oral bioavailability when given with liquid enteral formulas through feeding tubes in human patients (eg, 30%–80% bioavailable relative to direct oral administration).[1] In addition, enrofloxacin has decreased oral bioavailability in nursing kittens compared with chow-fed kittens.[2] Conversely, mitotane, which is quite lipophilic, is better absorbed with canned food or corn oil than in the fasted state in dogs.[3]

Oral bioavailability is also affected by patient factors, to include drug degradation by stomach acid, duodenal bacteria, or brush border enzymes; drug efflux by transporter pumps, and drug biotransformation by both the intestine and the liver, which together comprise the "first pass effect." The first pass effect can also lead to *increased* drug action if a drug or pro-drug is converted to an active metabolite; for example, codeine to morphine; enalapril to enalaprilat; and prednisone to prednisolone. The first pass effect is bypassed by IV, intramuscular, subcutaneous (SC), or transdermal drug administration.

Clinical application of bioavailability
- Bioavailability can be used to calculate drug dosages for different routes of administration
  - Oral dose = IV dose (reference route)/oral bioavailability
    - For a drug with 25% oral bioavailability, the oral dose will be 4 times that of the IV dose
  - Transdermal dose = oral dose (reference route)/transdermal bioavailability
    - For a drug with 10% transdermal bioavailability relative to oral administration, the transdermal dose would need to be 10 times that of the oral dose
    - An example of this is fluoxetine (10% transdermal bioavailability in cats); however, transdermal pluronic lethicin organogel (PLO) formulations that allowed higher doses led to skin irritation.[4]

Table 1
Mechanisms for low oral drug bioavailability

Sources of Low Oral Drug Bioavailability	Examples
Large molecule size	Insulin, erythropoietin
Highly polar drug (cannot cross lipid membranes of enterocytes)	Aminoglycosides, including oral neomycin Heparin Lidocaine
Drug binding to dietary cationic minerals (aluminum, calcium, zinc)	Fluoroquinolones Tetracyclines Theophylline Digoxin
Degradation by stomach acid, duodenal bacteria, or brush border enzymes	Salmon calcitonin: enzymatic degradation Erythromycin: acid degradation (rationale for enteric coated tablets)
High transporter efflux	Likely cyclosporine, rifampin, doxorubicin, and vincristine
High degree of intestinal and/or hepatic biotransformation to inactive metabolites	Oral budesonide, in humans

C_{max}

C_{max} is the highest (peak) plasma drug concentration that is reached after a given dose of a drug.

C_{max} is typically proportional to the dose, but may increase nonlinearly at higher doses (for example, with hydralazine dosing in dogs).[5] This phenomenon is typically due to saturation of clearance pathways, such as efflux transporters or cytochrome P450s. C_{max} also reflects the rate and extent of absorption, especially relative to the rate of elimination; for example, a drug with very slow absorption and a moderate rate of elimination will not accumulate and may have minimal pharmacodynamic effects (eg, ultralente insulin in the setting of ketoacidosis).

Clinical application of C_{max}
- C_{max} determines the magnitude of side effects for many drugs
  - Example: seizures after an IV bolus of lidocaine
- The ratio of drug C_{max} to bacterial MIC is used to optimize efficacy for some concentration-dependent antimicrobials.
  - Example: a C_{max}:MIC ratio of 10 or higher is targeted for aminoglycosides in human patients.[6]

Tmax

Tmax is the time at which the peak plasma drug concentration (C_{max}) is reached.

Tmax is affected primarily by the rate of drug absorption (relative to the rate of elimination). Both Tmax and C_{max} can be affected by food. For example, food given concomitantly with L-thyroxine in dogs delays Tmax and decreases C_{max} and overall bioavailability.[7] Therefore, L-thyroxine should ideally be given on an empty stomach, or at least in a consistent relationship to food in dogs; serum drug concentrations should also be monitored under the same feeding conditions as daily administration.

Clinical application of Tmax
- Tmax tells you when to expect many dose-dependent side effects.
  - Example: hypotension from hydralazine
  - Note: some peak drug effects can lag behind peak plasma concentrations (for example, with transmucosal buprenorphine in cats)[8]
- Tmax tells you when to draw a blood sample for monitoring peak drug concentrations
  - This is particularly important for drugs that are eliminated quickly, such as gabapentin in dogs (elimination half-life about 3.5 h),[9] because peak concentrations will be quite transient
  - For drugs that are eliminated slowly, such as potassium bromide, timing is much less important, because plasma drug concentrations will be fairly stable throughout a dosing interval.

Therapeutic Range (Therapeutic Window)

The therapeutic range (therapeutic window) is the range of plasma concentrations in which most patients have the desired drug effect with minimal toxicity.

For veterinary patients, the therapeutic range is often extrapolated from human studies and may not be well established in dogs or cats. The therapeutic index is the ratio between the upper (toxic) and lower (minimally effective) ends of the therapeutic range. If the therapeutic index is wide, this indicates a relatively safe drug. Conversely, a drug with a narrow therapeutic index has a small safety margin; for example, digoxin, with a therapeutic range of 0.8 to 1.2 ng/mL, has an unforgiving therapeutic index of less than 2.

For drugs with a narrow therapeutic range, therapeutic drug monitoring (measurement of plasma, serum, or whole-blood drug concentrations) can be used to optimize dose (**Table 2**). Therapeutic drug monitoring is also indicated for drugs that have variable bioavailability or clearance rates among individuals.

Area Under the Curve

The area under the curve (AUC) is the integrated area under the plasma drug concentration versus time curve.

AUC is a measure of drug exposure and is affected by dose, absorption, and clearance.

AUC is used to calculate drug bioavailability (for example, oral bioavailability = AUC (orally)/AUC IV). AUC (along with C_{max}) is also used to predict bioequivalence between a generic formulation and an established brand-name product with demonstrated efficacy. In addition, the ratio of drug AUC to bacterial MIC can be used to predict antimicrobial drug efficacy. For fluoroquinolone antibiotics, an AUC:MIC ratio of greater than 100 has been recommended for gram-negative infections, including *Pseudomonas aeruginosa* pneumonia in human patients.[14] This threshold is based on animal infection models and human clinical data; similar in vivo efficacy data have not been evaluated in dogs or cats.

Table 2
Drugs for which therapeutic drug monitoring is indicated

Drug	Timing	Reason for Monitoring
Thyroxine	Peak: 4–6 h after pill Want *high normal* levels	Variable concentrations at standard dosages[10]; due to differences in bioavailability and/or clearance
Phenobarbital	Timing not critical in most dogs[11] Long half-life relative to dosing interval	Variable hepatic biotransformation (degree of P450 induction)
Cyclosporine	Trough level before next dose	Variable bioavailability (CYP3A, p-glycoprotein)
Bromide	Timing not critical Long half-life relative to dosing interval	Variable renal clearance based on dietary chloride intake
Digoxin	6–8 h after dosing	Narrow therapeutic index Variable bioavailability (CYP3A, p-glycoprotein) Variable renal clearance
Theophylline	Extended release in dogs: Tmax 4–6 h after pill[12] Extended release in cats: Tmax 8 h after pill (Slo-bid and Theo-Dur)[13]	Variable bioavailability of extended release capsules
Gentamicin, amikacin	Peak: just after IV dosing, 30–40 min after SC dosing Trough: 24 h after dosing	Narrow therapeutic index C_{max} correlates with bacterial kill Trough (C_{min}) correlates with nephrotoxicity

Volume of Distribution (Vd)

Volume of distribution (Vd) is the ratio between the total amount of drug administered and the resulting plasma drug concentrations.

Vd can be thought of as a "patient beaker" into which you are pouring the drug. A low Vd suggests that drug distribution may be limited to the plasma space. This drug distribution is seen with highly protein-bound drugs such as cefovecin (Vd ~0.1 L/kg in dogs and cats; Convenia label). In this case, bound drug remains in the plasma space and acts as a drug depot, while free drug can still reach target sites of infection.

Conversely, a high Vd indicates extensive distribution of total drug out of the plasma. This distribution of total drug is desirable if it reflects drug that is distributed to the interstitial and intracellular spaces, because the drug is likely to reach the target receptor, site of inflammation, or source of infection. However, a large Vd does not necessarily mean that the drug is distributed to the desired target site. Very high Vd estimates (>1.0 L/kg) can result from drug binding in off-target tissues, such as bone or skeletal muscle. An example of this is digoxin, which is extensively bound to skeletal muscle and has a Vd of greater than 10 L/kg in dogs.[15]

Clinical application of Vd
- Vd can be used to determine the loading dose of a drug
  - Loading dose in mg/kg = desired plasma concentration (mg/L) × Vd in L/kg
  - Example: for a phenobarbital target concentration of 30 ug/mL (=30 mg/L), with a Vd of 0.75 L/kg,[16] the calculated IV loading dose is 22.5 mg/kg.

Clearance

Clearance is the volume of plasma that is cleared of drug over time.

Clearance reflects all routes of drug elimination, including hepatic biotransformation, biliary excretion, glomerular filtration, and renal tubular secretion. Clearance mechanisms are common sites of drug interactions (see article "Adverse drug reactions in veterinary patients associated with drug transporters" elsewhere in this issue). In addition, decreased hepatic or renal function can lead to impaired drug clearance and the need for drug dose adjustment.

In human patients with significant hepatocellular dysfunction, drugs that are cleared by the liver and have relatively narrow therapeutic ranges merit dosage reduction (**Table 3**). These same adjustments are likely to apply to dogs and cats with portosystemic shunts, acute hepatocellular necrosis, severe hepatic lipidosis, or acquired cirrhosis, although few studies have been performed in veterinary species.

In patients with renal insufficiency, dosages of renally cleared drugs, especially those with narrow therapeutic ranges, should also be adjusted. Drug dosage reductions are often made in human patients when creatinine clearance values are less than ~0.7 mL/min/kg (depending on the drug). Although this is equivalent to a serum creatinine of 3.5 mg/dL in cats,[17,18] minimal data are available in dogs, and lack equivalent dose adjustment studies are lacking in both species. Until better studies are available, only human data can be extrapolated; empiric recommendations are given in **Table 4**.

Elimination Half-Life

Elimination half-life is the time it takes for plasma concentrations of a drug to decrease by 50%.

Elimination half-life is important for determining the time to reach steady-state (stable or equilibrium) plasma concentrations. Time to steady state takes approximately

Table 3
Suggested drug dosage adjustments in hepatic failure

Drug	Recommended Adjustment
Chloramphenicol	Avoid if possible If used, monitor CBC for bone marrow suppression Consider reducing dosage, but accurate guidelines not available
Diazepam or midazolam	Use with caution Consider using 25%–50% of standard dosages
Furosemide	Use with caution Hypokalemia may precipitate hepatic encephalopathy Consider substituting spironolactone/hydrochlothiazide when treating ascites
Lidocaine	Avoid or reduce dosage (eg, by ~50%)
Metronidazole	Reduce total daily dose to one-third of standard anti-anaerobic dosage, and dose once daily
Phenobarbital	Avoid or discontinue If using for seizures from congenital portosystemic shunting, consider starting at 25%–50% of standard dosages, or choose potassium bromide
Propranolol	Decrease daily dosage by 50% or more Monitor heart rate and blood pressure
Theophylline	Reduce oral dose (eg, by ~50%) Measure serum theophylline concentrations

Data from Recommendations for humans by the World Health Organization, WHO model formulary, 2008. Available at: http://whqlibdoc.who.int/publications/2009/9789241547659_eng.pdf. Accessed December 10, 2012.

5 elimination half-lives for any drug. Note that steady-state plasma drug concentrations may or may not be in the therapeutic range, depending on what dosage you choose. Elimination half-life is also important for determining dosing frequency, which is based on both the elimination half-life and the therapeutic range (ie, the allowable change in plasma concentrations between doses). Finally, elimination half-life determines the time when a given drug or toxin will be eliminated from the body after administration or exposure.

Clinical applications of elimination half-life include the following:
- Elimination half-life determines time when steady-state serum drug concentrations can be measured
  - Example: the elimination half-life of modified cyclosporine (ie, the microemulsion formulation found in Atopica and Neoral) is 6 to 12 hours in dogs[25,26]; therefore, steady state should be reached in $5 \times 12 = 60$ hours, so steady-state whole blood concentrations can be measured in 2.5 to 3 days.
- Elimination half-life determines dosing frequency
  - Example: the elimination half-life of levetiracetam as a single agent in dogs is about 4 hours[27]; with a proposed therapeutic range of 5 to 30 μg/mL in humans (ARUP Laboratories, Salt Lake City, UT), this requires dosing every 8 hours.
  - In addition, concurrent administration of phenobarbital shortens the half-life of levetiracetam further, to about 2 hours,[27] which could lead to subtherapeutic levetiracetam concentrations during an 8-h dosing interval and needs further evaluation.

Table 4
Empiric recommendations for drug dosage adjustment in dogs and cats with renal failure

Drug	Standard Dosage	CL Creatinine of 0.4–0.7 mL/kg/min (30–50 mL/min in Humans) Roughly a Serum Creatinine of 2.3–4.0 mg/dL in Cats[17-19]	CL Creatinine of 0.15–0.4 mL/kg/min (10–30 mL/min in Humans) Roughly a Serum Creatinine of 4.9–5.5 mg/dL[17,20]	CL Creatinine of <0.15 mL/kg/min (<10 mL/min in Humans) Roughly a Serum Creatinine of 8.5 mg/dL[17]
Amikacin[21]	15 mg/kg q24h	q36–48h Avoid if possible	q48h Avoid if possible	Not recommended
Amphotericin B	1 mg/kg IV 3 times weekly	Use liposomal formulation (AmBisome; less nephrotoxic)[22]	Use liposomal formulation; only with careful monitoring	Avoid if possible
Atenolol	0.25 mg/kg q12h	No change to 50% of total daily dose	50% of total daily dose	25% of total daily dose
Benazepril	0.5 mg/kg q12h	No change	Start at 50% of total daily dose	Start at 50% of total daily dose
Cefazolin	20 mg/kg q8h	q12h	q12h	q24h
Cefotetan[23]	30 mg/kg SC q12h	No change	q24h	q48h
Enalapril	0.5 mg/kg q12h	No change recommended in humans[a]	Start at 50% of total daily dose	Start at 50% of total daily dose
Enrofloxacin	5 mg/kg q24h	Presumption is to extend dosing interval (as for ciprofloxacin in humans); substitute less retinotoxic fluoroquinolones such as marbofloxacin	Not recommended in cats due to risk of retinotoxicity	Not recommended in cats due to risk of retinotoxicity

(continued on next page)

Table 4
(continued)

Drug	Standard Dosage	CL Creatinine of 0.4–0.7 mL/kg/min (30–50 mL/min in Humans) Roughly a Serum Creatinine of 2.3–4.0 mg/dL in Cats[17–19]	CL Creatinine of 0.15–0.4 mL/kg/min (10–30 mL/min in Humans) Roughly a Serum Creatinine of 4.9–5.5 mg/dL[17,20]	CL Creatinine of <0.15 mL/kg/min (<10 mL/min in Humans) Roughly a Serum Creatinine of 8.5 mg/dL[17]
Famotidine	1 mg/kg q12h	q24h	q24h	q24h
Fluconazole	5 mg/kg q12h	50% of total daily dose	50% of total daily dose	50% of total daily dose
Fluoxetine	1–2 mg/kg q24h	No change	No change	50% of total daily dose
Gabapentin	10 mg/kg q8h (starting dose)	6 mg/kg q12h	6 mg/kg q4h	3–4 mg/kg q24h
Gentamicin[21]	6–8 mg/kg q24h	q36–48h Avoid if possible	q48h Avoid if possible	Not recommended
Levetiracetam	20 mg/kg q8h	50% of total daily dose	30%–50% of total daily dose	30%–50% of total daily dose
Metoclopramide	1–2 mg/kg/d CRI	50% of total daily dose	50% of total daily dose	25%–50% of total daily dose
Spironolactone	1.0 mg/kg q12h	No change	No change	Not recommended
Trimethoprim/ sulfamethoxazole	15 mg/kg q12h	No change Avoid sulfadiazine due to higher risk of crystalluria	50% dose reduction q12h Avoid sulfadiazine	Not recommended

[a] Studies in dogs with renal impairment (Creatinine clearance [Clcr] of 1.7 mL/kg/min) showed an increase in AUC by 80% for active enalaprilat.[24]
Data from University of Wisconsin Hospital and Clinics Clinical Directive for Renal Function-Based Dose Adjustments in Adults, 2009. Available at: http://www. uwhealth.org/files/uwhealth/docs/antimicrobial/Renal_Function_Based_Dose_Adjustment_In_Adults_Protocol_2010.pdf. Accessed December 10, 2012.

- Elimination half-life determines time for washout of a drug or toxin
  - For example, to switch from clomipramine to fluoxetine in a dog with behavioral anxiety, it is important to wait for complete washout of clomipramine, because this drug is contraindicated in combination with selective serotonin reuptake inhibitors.[28]
  - The washout period would therefore be 5 elimination half-lives for both clomipramine and any active metabolites.
  - With a t½ of up to 16 hours for clomipramine and 3 hours for the active metabolite desmethylclomipramine in dogs,[29] washout would be 5 × 16 hours, or between 3 and 4 days before fluoxetine could be started.

Table 5
Phase I drug biotransformation pathways

Enzymes	Activities	Example Substrates and Clinical Relevance
Cytochrome P450s	Oxidation Reduction Hydrolysis	CYP1A2: Clearance of caffeine, theophylline, pentoxifylline in humans; bioactivation of environmental carcinogens. CYP1A2 is polymorphic in dogs[30] CYP2B11: Clearance of propofol, ketamine, and midazolam in dogs[31,32] CYP2B11 seems to be polymorphic in dogs[32] CYP3A family: Clearance of midazolam and presumably cyclosporine in dogs[33,34] CYP3A is inhibited by ketoconazole in dogs and cats[34,35]
Flavin monooxygenases	Oxidation	Methimazole is a substrate (shown in humans and dogs)[36]
Alcohol dehydrogenase	Converts alcohols to aldehydes	Important for ethanol and ethylene glycol metabolism Inhibitory target for 4-methylpyrazole
Aldehyde dehydrogenases	Convert aldehydes to carboxylic acids	Important for ethanol and ethylene glycol clearance Inhibited by chloramphenicol, and by disulfiram (Antabuse; used to treat alcoholism)
Monoamine oxidases	Inactivate bioamines by converting them to aldehydes	Endogenous substrates include epinephrine, norepinephrine, dopamine, and serotonin Inhibitory target for MAO inhibitors, such as L-deprenyl and amitraz
Plasma esterases	Hydrolyze ester bonds	Pseudocholinesterases inactivate succinylcholine and other neuromuscular blocking drugs
Epoxide hydrolases	Break down reactive epoxide metabolites	Involved in the detoxification of phenytoin, carbamazepine, and possibly phenobarbital[37]

Biotransformation

Biotransformation is the chemical modification of a drug, typically by phase I or phase II enzymes.

Biotransformation pathways have evolved to detoxify foreign chemicals and to facilitate excretion. Most orally absorbed xenobiotics require some degree of biotransformation because drugs must be somewhat lipophilic to be absorbed across intestinal membranes. However, lipophilic compounds need to be biotransformed to more polar derivatives to be excreted by renal and biliary transporters. Although the liver is a major site of phase I and phase II biotransformation, these drug metabolism pathways are also present in the intestine, lung, kidney, brain, adrenal, and other sites.

Phase I enzymes modify drugs through oxidation, reduction, or hydrolysis (**Table 5**). Cytochrome P450s are a major group of phase I enzymes. P450s are found in the endoplasmic reticulum of cells; the endoplasmic reticulum forms microsomes when isolated from cells in vitro, thus the term "microsomal P450s." Cytochrome P450s usually inactivate compounds and can also facilitate phase II biotransformation by creating sites that provide a "handle" (such as a hydroxyl group, –OH) for conjugation. Less commonly, cytochrome P450s can bioactivate compounds, for example, for

Table 6
Phase II drug conjugation pathways

Enzymes (Conjugated Molecule)	Features	Example Substrates
UDP-glucuronosyltranferases (glucuronide)	Cats have inactive pseudogene for UGT1A6[40]	Acetaminophen Aspirin
Glutathione-S-transferases (glutathione)	Multiple GST families Some dogs lack GST-θ expression[41] GST-θ variant associated with lymphoma risk in dogs[42]	Environmental carcinogens Insecticides and herbicides Acrolein (metabolite of cyclophosphamide) Doxorubicin Felbamate
Sulfotransferases (sulfate)	Multiple SULT families	Methimazole Acetaminophen Dopamine Terbutaline Thyroxine intermediates
N-acetyltransferases (acetyl group)	Not expressed in dogs (lack NAT1 and NAT2 genes)[43]	Sulfonamide antimicrobials Hydralazine Procainamide Dapsone
Thiopurine methyltransferases (methyl group)	Low activity in cats; likely cause of bone marrow suppression at standard azathioprine dosages in cats[44] Ninefold range in RBC activity in dogs[45]; but low RBC activity was not found in dogs with azathioprine myelosuppression[46]	Azathioprine metabolites
Glycine N-acyltransferases (glycine)	Mitochondrial enzyme Not well characterized in dogs or cats	Detoxification of benzoate, xylene, salicylate[47]

pro-drugs such as enalaprilat (biotransformed to enalapril), codeine (converted to morphine), and azathioprine (metabolized to 6-mercaptopurine). Cytochrome P450s can occasionally render drugs more toxic. For example, CYP2E1 converts acetaminophen to its reactive metabolite, NAPQI, which leads to dose-dependent hepatotoxicity.

Phase II enzymes result in the addition (via a covalent bond) of an extra group to the drug **(Table 6)**. These drug conjugates are usually inactive and are rendered more polar to facilitate excretion. Classic examples of this are glucuronide conjugation of acetaminophen (impaired in cats) and N-acetylation of sulfonamide antimicrobials (absent in dogs). Conversely, however, drug conjugation sometimes can increase the toxicity of xenobiotics, such as environmental carcinogens. An example of this is the bladder carcinogen 4-aminobiphenyl, which is found in tobacco smoke. 4-Aminobiphenyl is bioactivated after glucuronide conjugation in both humans and dogs, leading to a reactive product that forms DNA adducts in the bladder mucosa.[38] Genetic variability in the efficiency of glucuronidation is a bladder cancer risk factor in humans[39]; however, this has not been explored in dogs.

SUMMARY

Pharmacokinetic data are often available for the drugs that are prescribed in dogs and are sometimes available in cats. This information can be used in many practical ways, to include dosage extrapolations from one route to another, timing of blood sample collection for therapeutic drug monitoring, optimizing therapy with concentration-dependent antimicrobials, understanding marketing brochures for new drugs, and adjusting drug dosages based on impaired liver or kidney function. As more is learned about specific biotransformation pathways involved in the clearance of commonly used drugs, as well as breed differences in these pathways, these data may also be used to tailor drug therapy more effectively for individual patients.

REFERENCES

1. Mimoz O, Binter V, Jacolot A, et al. Pharmacokinetics and absolute bioavailability of ciprofloxacin administered through a nasogastric tube with continuous enteral feeding to critically ill patients. Intensive Care Med 1998;24:1047–51.
2. Seguin MA, Papich MG, Sigle KJ, et al. Pharmacokinetics of enrofloxacin in neonatal kittens. Am J Vet Res 2004;65:350–6.
3. Watson AD, Rijnberk A, Moolenaar AJ. Systemic availability of o,p'-DDD in normal dogs, fasted and fed, and in dogs with hyperadrenocorticism. Res Vet Sci 1987; 43:160–5.
4. Ciribassi J, Luescher A, Pasloske KS, et al. Comparative bioavailability of fluoxetine after transdermal and oral administration to healthy cats. Am J Vet Res 2003;64:994–8.
5. Semple HA, Tam YK, Coutts RT. Hydralazine pharmacokinetics and interaction with food: an evaluation of the dog as an animal model. Pharm Res 1990;7:274–9.
6. Rea RS, Capitano B. Optimizing use of aminoglycosides in the critically ill. Semin Respir Crit Care Med 2007;28:596–603.
7. Le Traon G, Burgaud S, Horspool LJ. Pharmacokinetics of total thyroxine in dogs after administration of an oral solution of levothyroxine sodium. J Vet Pharmacol Ther 2008;31:95–101.
8. Robertson SA, Lascelles BD, Taylor PM, et al. PK-PD modeling of buprenorphine in cats: intravenous and oral transmucosal administration. J Vet Pharmacol Ther 2005;28:453–60.

9. Kukanich B, Cohen RL. Pharmacokinetics of oral gabapentin in greyhound dogs. Vet J 2011;187:133–5.

10. Nachreiner RF, Refsal KR. Radioimmunoassay monitoring of thyroid hormone concentrations in dogs on thyroid replacement therapy: 2,674 cases (1985-1987). J Am Vet Med Assoc 1992;201:623–9.

11. Levitski RE, Trepanier LA. Effect of timing of blood collection on serum phenobarbital concentrations in dogs with epilepsy. J Am Vet Med Assoc 2000;217: 200–4.

12. Bach JE, Kukanich B, Papich MG, et al. Evaluation of the bioavailability and pharmacokinetics of two extended-release theophylline formulations in dogs. J Am Vet Med Assoc 2004;224:1113–9.

13. Dye JA, McKiernan BC, Jones SD, et al. Sustained-release theophylline pharmacokinetics in the cat. J Vet Pharmacol Ther 1989;12:133–40.

14. Wispelwey B. Clinical implications of pharmacokinetics and pharmacodynamics of fluoroquinolones. Clin Infect Dis 2005;41(Suppl 2):S127–35.

15. Button C, Gross DR, Johnston JT, et al. Pharmacokinetics, bioavailability, and dosage regimens of digoxin in dogs. Am J Vet Res 1980;41:1230–7.

16. Plumb D. Veterinary drug handbook. 7th edition. Ames (IA): Iowa State University Press; 2011.

17. Miyamoto K. Clinical application of plasma clearance of iohexol on feline patients. J Feline Med Surg 2001;3:143–7.

18. Sox EM, Chiotti R, Goldstein RE. Use of gadolinium diethylene triamine pentaacetic acid, as measured by ELISA, in the determination of glomerular filtration rates in cats. J Feline Med Surg 2010;12:738–45.

19. Haller M, Rohner K, Muller W, et al. Single-injection inulin clearance for routine measurement of glomerular filtration rate in cats. J Feline Med Surg 2003;5: 175–81.

20. Heiene R, Reynolds BS, Bexfield NH, et al. Estimation of glomerular filtration rate via 2- and 4-sample plasma clearance of iohexol and creatinine in clinically normal cats. Am J Vet Res 2009;70:176–85.

21. Nayak-Rao S. Aminoglycoside use in renal failure. Indian J Nephrol 2010;20: 121–4.

22. Bekersky I, Boswell GW, Hiles R, et al. Safety and toxicokinetics of intravenous liposomal amphotericin B (AmBisome) in beagle dogs. Pharm Res 1999;16: 1694–701.

23. Smith BR, LeFrock JL, Thyrum PT, et al. Cefotetan pharmacokinetics in volunteers with various degrees of renal function. Antimicrob Agents Chemother 1986;29: 887–93.

24. Lefebvre HP, Laroute V, Concordet D, et al. Effects of renal impairment on the disposition of orally administered enalapril, benazepril, and their active metabolites. J Vet Intern Med 1999;13:21–7.

25. Allenspach K, Rufenacht S, Sauter S, et al. Pharmacokinetics and clinical efficacy of cyclosporine treatment of dogs with steroid-refractory inflammatory bowel disease. J Vet Intern Med 2006;20:239–44.

26. Radwanski NE, Cerundolo R, Shofer FS, et al. Effects of powdered whole grapefruit and metoclopramide on the pharmacokinetics of cyclosporine in dogs. Am J Vet Res 2011;72:687–93.

27. Moore SA, Munana KR, Papich MG, et al. The pharmacokinetics of levetiracetam in healthy dogs concurrently receiving phenobarbital. J Vet Pharmacol Ther 2011; 34:31–4.

28. Gillman PK. Tricyclic antidepressant pharmacology and therapeutic drug interactions updated. Br J Pharmacol 2007;151:737–48.
29. Hewson CJ, Conlon PD, Luescher UA, et al. The pharmacokinetics of clomipramine and desmethylclomipramine in dogs: parameter estimates following a single oral dose and 28 consecutive daily oral doses of clomipramine. J Vet Pharmacol Ther 1998;21:214–22.
30. Scherr MC, Lourenco GJ, Albuquerque DM, et al. Polymorphism of cytochrome P450 A2 (CYP1A2) in pure and mixed breed dogs. J Vet Pharmacol Ther 2011; 34:184–6.
31. Baratta MT, Zaya MJ, White JA, et al. Canine CYP2B11 metabolizes and is inhibited by anesthetic agents often co-administered in dogs. J Vet Pharmacol Ther 2010;33:50–5.
32. Hay-Kraus B, Greenblatt D, Venkatakrishnan K, et al. Evidence of propofol hydroxylation by cytochrome P4502B11 in canine liver microsomes: breed and gender differences. Xenobiotica 2000;30:575–88.
33. D'Mello A, Venkataramanan R, Satake M, et al. Pharmacokinetics of the cyclosporine-ketoconazole interaction in dogs. Res Commun Chem Pathol Pharmacol 1989;64:441–54.
34. Kuroha M, Azumano A, Kuze Y, et al. Effect of multiple dosing of ketoconazole on pharmacokinetics of midazolam, a cytochrome P450 3A substrate in beagle dogs. Drug Metab Dispos 2002;30:63–8.
35. McAnulty JF, Lensmeyer GL. The effects of ketoconazole on the pharmacokinetics of cyclosporine A in cats. Vet Surg 1999;28:448–55.
36. Lattard V, Longin-Sauvageon C, Lachuer J, et al. Cloning, sequencing, and tissue-dependent expression of flavin-containing monooxygenase (FMO) 1 and FMO3 in the dog. Drug Metab Dispos 2002;30:119–28.
37. Santos NA, Medina WS, Martins NM, et al. Involvement of oxidative stress in the hepatotoxicity induced by aromatic antiepileptic drugs. Toxicol In Vitro 2008;22: 1820–4.
38. Kadlubar FF, Miller JA, Miller EC. Hepatic microsomal N-glucuronidation and nucleic acid binding of N-hydroxy arylamines in relation to urinary bladder carcinogenesis. Cancer Res 1977;37:805–14.
39. Cui X, Lu X, Hiura M, et al. Association of genotypes of carcinogen-metabolizing enzymes and smoking status with bladder cancer in a Japanese population. Environ Health Prev Med 2013;18(2):136–42.
40. Court MH, Greenblatt DJ. Molecular genetic basis for deficient acetaminophen glucuronidation by cats: UGT1A6 is a pseudogene, and evidence for reduced diversity of expressed hepatic UGT1A isoforms. Pharmacogenetics 2000;10: 355–69.
41. Watanabe T, Ohashi Y, Kosaka T, et al. Expression of the theta class GST isozyme, YdfYdf, in low GST dogs. Arch Toxicol 2006;80:250–7.
42. Ginn J, Sacco J, Wong YY, et al. Positive association between a glutathione-S-transferase polymorphism and lymphoma in dogs. Vet Comp Oncol June 2, 2013. [Epub ahead of print].
43. Trepanier LA, Ray K, Winand NJ, et al. Cytosolic arylamine N-acetyltransferase (NAT) deficiency in the dog and other canids due to an absence of NAT genes. Biochem Pharmacol 1997;54:73–80.
44. White SD, Rosychuk RA, Outerbridge CA, et al. Thiopurine methyltransferase in red blood cells of dogs, cats, and horses. J Vet Intern Med 2000;14: 499–502.

45. Kidd LB, Salavaggione OE, Szumlanski CL, et al. Thiopurine methyltransferase activity in red blood cells of dogs. J Vet Intern Med 2004;18:214–8.
46. Rodriguez DB, Mackin A, Easley R, et al. Relationship between red blood cell thiopurine methyltransferase activity and myelotoxicity in dogs receiving azathioprine. J Vet Intern Med 2004;18:339–45.
47. van der Sluis R, Badenhorst CP, van der Westhuizen FH, et al. Characterisation of the influence of genetic variations on the enzyme activity of a recombinant human glycine N-acyltransferase. Gene 2013;515:447–53.

Canine Cytochrome P-450 Pharmacogenetics

Michael H. Court, BVSc, PhD

KEYWORDS

- Dog • Canine • Genetic polymorphism • Cytochrome P-450 • Pharmacokinetics

KEY POINTS

- Polymorphisms in genes encoding CYP enzymes could explain adverse drug effects or therapeutic failure in canine patients.
- A premature stop codon mutation in CYP1A2 is commonly found in certain dog breeds, including Beagle and Irish wolfhound.
- Although the CYP1A2 premature stop codon has shown large effects on the pharmacokinetics of some experimental compounds, effects on commonly used clinical drugs is currently unknown.
- Polymorphisms also exist in genes encoding canine CYP2C41, CYP2E1, CYP2D15, and CYP3A12 that have the potential to impact the metabolism of a large number of different drugs.
- Anesthetic drug hypersensitivity in Greyhounds may be the result of a genetic variant affecting canine CYP2B11 expression or function.

INTRODUCTION

The cytochrome P-450 (CYP) drug-metabolizing enzymes are critical to the efficient elimination of many drugs used in clinical practice. Unfortunately in humans, and probably in all species of veterinary importance, there is considerable interindividual variability in the activity of these enzymes.[1] Consequently, for a given drug dosage the effect can range from undetectable or suboptimal (with high enzyme activity, high drug clearance, and low plasma levels) to excessive or toxic (with low enzyme activity, low drug clearance, and high plasma levels). Causes of this variability can include concurrent exposure to CYP enzyme inhibitors or inducers in the diet or from coadministered medications (previously reviewed[2]). Genetic variation is also a well-established

Disclosures: This work was supported by funds provided by the William R. Jones Endowed Chair in Veterinary Medicine at Washington State University. There are no conflicts of interest to report.
Department of Veterinary Clinical Sciences, College of Veterinary Medicine, Washington State University, 100 Grimes Way, Pullman, WA 99164, USA
E-mail address: Michael.Court@vetmed.wsu.edu

cause of CYP activity variability in humans, and current evidence suggests that it may be equally important in veterinary species, including dogs.[1] Consequently, clinical assays for CYP gene variants that significantly impact drug disposition could be a useful tool to enable rational drug selection and dosage for the individual patient. This article reviews the current state of knowledge regarding the dog CYPs focusing on potentially clinically important genetic variants that could influence drug efficacy and toxicity.

DOG-HUMAN CYP SIMILARITIES AND DIFFERENCES

Much of the available published data on the CYPs so far concern the human CYPs. Indeed, the US Food and Drug Administration requires detailed label information regarding the involvement of specific human CYPs in the metabolism of all newly approved drugs intended for use in humans. Although much of the information can be applied in a general fashion to the dog CYPs, it is becoming increasingly apparent that there are important differences in the metabolism of drugs by human and dog CYPs, much of which have yet to be determined. Specific examples of some of the known similarities and differences are discussed next.

CYP Substrate Specificity

Table 1 lists common CYP drug substrates in humans compared with dogs. The CYPs are named according to gene sequence similarity and grouped according to family (number), subfamily (letter), and unique gene product (number), as in the canine CYP2B11 gene (family, 2; subfamily, B; 11th gene identified). Because of significant species differences in gene sequence of these enzymes, each species tends to have their unique CYP names, although orthologs (genes derived from the same ancestral gene that diverged after speciation) are found in most species. For example, CYP2B11 is considered to be the canine ortholog of human CYP2B6.[3,4] Orthologs also tend to have roughly similar substrate specificities. For example, human CYP2B6 and canine CYP2B11 metabolize propofol.[4,5] However, significant species differences exist. For example, midazolam is metabolized exclusively by human CYP3A4 and CYP3A5 (but not by human CYP2B6), whereas dog CYP2B11 (and not CYP3A12) primarily metabolizes midazolam.[6] Similarly, dog CYP1A2 and dog CYP2A13 metabolize phenacetin,[7,8] whereas only human CYP1A2 (and not human CYP2A6) metabolizes this drug. Although most dog CYPs have unique names, three of the drug-metabolizing CYPs (CYP1A1, CYP1A2, and CYP2E1) have identical names to those found in other mammalian species, in part because they have relatively conserved gene sequences between species, and in part because their naming preceded the convention to give unique names to the drug-metabolizing CYPs in different species.

CYP Abundance

Apart from differences in catalytic properties between dog and human CYPs, these enzymes also differ in the relative amount of each family and subfamily between dogs and humans. **Fig. 1** shows the distribution of the different CYPs in liver and small intestinal mucosa of human[9,10] and dog.[11] The liver has the highest content of drug-metabolizing CYPs and is the most important organ for CYP-mediated drug elimination. The small intestine also has a high specific content of certain CYPs located within the mucosa and serves to decrease absorption of intact (unmetabolized) drugs thereby limiting systemic availability of orally administered drugs. Similarities between dog and human are apparent in that the CYP3A subfamily enzymes are the predominant isoforms in liver and intestines of both species. However, the CYP2D subfamily

Table 1
Examples of drugs that are known substrates for specific human[a] or dog[b] CYPs

Human CYP	Substrates	Dog CYP	Substrates
CYP1A2	Caffeine Phenacetin Tacrine Theophylline	CYP1A2	Caffeine Phenacetin Theophylline
CYP2A6	Nicotine	CYP2A13	Phenacetin
CYP2B6	Bupropion Efavirenz Propofol	CYP2B11	Atipamezole Diclofenac Ketamine Medetomidine Midazolam Propofol Temazepam
CYP2C8	Amodiaquine	CYP2C21/CYP2C41	Diclofenac
CYP2C9	Diclofenac Tolbutamide S-warfarin		
CYP2C19	Omeprazole S-mephenytoin		
CYP2D6	Bufuralol Codeine Debrisoquine Dextromethorphan	CYP2D15	Celecoxib Debrisoquine (poor) Desipramine Dextromethorphan Imipramine
CYP2E1	Chlorzoxazone	CYP2E1	Chlorzoxazone
CYP3A4	Midazolam Triazolam Terfenadine Nifedipine	CYP3A12	Diazepam Diclofenac Eplerenone Imatinib Midazolam

Both sources also list other dog and human CYP substrates, inhibitors, and inducers.

[a] *Data from* P450 Drug Interaction Table. Indiana University Department of Medicine. 2009. Available at: http://medicine.iupui.edu/clinpharm/ddis/table.aspx. Accessed April 20, 2013.

[b] *Data from* Martinez MN, Antonovic L, Court M, et al. Challenges in exploring the cytochrome P450 system as a source of variation in canine drug pharmacokinetics. L Drug Metab Rev 2013;45(2):218–30.

enzyme CYP2D15 is more highly expressed (as a percentage of total CYPs) in the livers of dogs versus CYP2D6 in humans. Furthermore, the CYP2B subfamily enzyme CYP2B11 is more highly expressed in both livers and intestines of dogs than CYP2B6 in human livers and intestines. This difference could be a consequence of the many genetic mutations that have been associated with the CYP2D6 and CYP2B6 genes in humans. A clinical consequence is that drugs metabolized by CYP2D or CYP2B may have lower systemic levels in dogs than in humans.

CANINE CYPS WITH KNOWN GENETIC POLYMORPHISM

Table 2 summarizes published data regarding known genetic polymorphisms in the canine drug-metabolizing CYP enzymes including variant description, allele frequencies, and effects of the variant on enzyme function in vitro and in vivo.

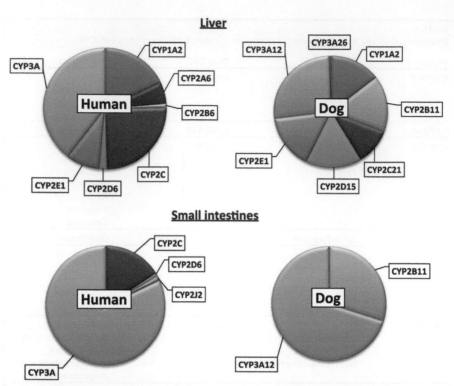

Fig. 1. Comparison of relative CYP isoform protein levels in dog and human liver and small intestines. Protein amounts were determined by quantitative immunoblotting for human liver[10] and intestines[9] or by quantitative mass spectrometry for Beagle dog tissues.[11] Note that CYP2A forms were not assayed in dog tissues, and CYPs other than CYP2B11 and CYP3A12 were below the detection level in dog intestines.

CYP1A2 Premature Stop Codon (CYP1A2stop) Polymorphism

The most comprehensively studied canine CYP genetic polymorphism is the premature stop codon mutation (c.1117C>T; R373X) located in the coding region of the CYP1A2 gene that results in complete loss of hepatic CYP1A2 protein and associated enzyme activity.[12,13] This mutation was discovered independently by two Japanese pharmaceutical companies during preclinical testing of two unrelated investigational compounds (YM-64227[12] and AC3933[13]) that showed highly polymorphic pharmacokinetics of these compounds in their Beagle dog colonies. Both groups used genetic testing to screen a large number of their Beagle dog colonies and found that from 11% to 17% of their dogs had the homozygous mutant genotype and consequently did not express functional CYP1A2.[12,13] The effect on the plasma drug levels of the investigational drugs was large with up to 17 times increased levels in deficient dogs (**Fig. 2**).[20,21] However, animals that had at least one normal CYP1A2 copy (heterozygotes) did not have substantially different drug levels from the wild-type dogs. Several other investigational compounds including GTS-21[22] and BTP-2[23] have also been associated with variable CYP1A2 metabolism in Beagles.

The effect of this polymorphism on the pharmacokinetics and effects of clinically used drugs is unclear. In vitro studies[8] using liver microsomes from CYP1A2-deficient and -expressing dogs indicated that phenacetin and tacrine (both selectively metabolized by human CYP1A2) were more slowly metabolized in deficient livers.

Table 2
Summary of known canine CYP genetic polymorphisms

Enzyme	Genetic Variant	Variant Allele Frequency	In Vitro Effect	In Vivo Effect
CYP1A2	SNP c.1117C> T causing premature stop codon mutation at amino acid position 373 (R373X)	6% in 99 mixed-breed dogs from Brazil; 38% in 214 Beagles from Japan; see **Fig. 3** for complete numbers	No functional enzyme	~ 50% lower phenacetin clearance after oral administration; no difference in phenacetin clearance after intravenous administration
CYP2C41	Partial or complete gene deletion	Gene absent in 24 of 28 (86%) dogs (Beagles and mixed breed)	No functional enzyme	Unknown
CYP2D15	S186G, I250F, I307V (WT2)	Unknown	Lower bufuralol hydroxylation than V1,*2 and *3; dextromethorphan demethylation and celecoxib hydroxylation same as for V1,*2 and *3	Unknown
	S186G, I250F, I307V, I338V, K407E (V1)	Unknown	No effect	Unknown
	S186G (CYP2D15*2)	Unknown	No effect	Unknown
	I250F, I307V (CYP2D15*3)	Unknown	No effect	Unknown
CYP2E1	Y485D	15% in 100 mixed-breed dogs; 19% in 13 Beagles	No effect	Unknown
CYP3A12	T309S, R421K, K422E, N423K, M452T	Unknown	No effect	Unknown

Data from Refs.[12–19]

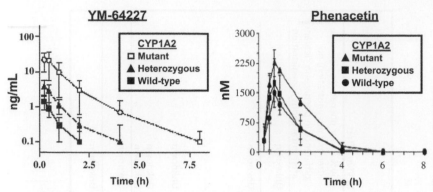

Fig. 2. Effect of the CYP1A2 premature stop codon mutation (R373X) on the pharmacokinetics of the investigational compound YM-64227 (*left*) and the analgesic drug phenacetin (*right*) after oral administration to genotyped Beagle dogs. The effect of the CYP1A2 premature stop codon on YM-64227 (about 25 times greater mean plasma area under the curve) was much greater than on phenacetin (about two times greater area under the curve). (YM-64227 *Data from* Tenmizu D, Noguchi K, Kamimura H, et al. The canine CYP1A2 deficiency polymorphism dramatically affects the pharmacokinetics of 4-cyclohexyl-1-ethyl-7-methylpyrido 2,3-D -pyrimidine-2-(1H)-one (YM-64227), a phosphodiesterase type 4 inhibitor. Drug Metab Dispos 2006;34(5):800; Phenacetin *Data from* Whiterock VJ, Morgan DG, Lentz KA, et al. Phenacetin pharmacokinetics in CYP1A2-deficient beagle dogs. Drug Metab Dispos 2012;40(2):228–31.)

However, other (human selective) CYP1A2 substrates including caffeine and melatonin were unaffected by the deficiency, implying that dog CYP1A2 does not selectively metabolize these latter drugs (unlike human CYP1A2). A recent study of phenacetin pharmacokinetics following oral and intravenous administration to CYP1A2 genotyped Beagles[15] showed about twofold higher phenacetin exposure (based on area under the plasma concentration time curve) after oral administration in CYP1A2-deficient dogs, but there were much smaller (nonsignificant) differences in phenacetin levels after intravenous exposure. The authors concluded that phenacetin was not a selective or robust in vivo probe for CYP1A2 probably because of metabolism of phenacetin by other enzymes (eg, canine CYP1A1 or canine CYP2A13). These findings indicate that the effect of CYP1A2stop on a particular drug depends on the degree of importance of canine CYP1A2 in clearance and cannot be extrapolated directly from human data.

The prevalence of CYP1A2stop seems to vary considerably between and within dog breeds. Apart from research colony Beagle dogs in Japan,[12,13] several other studies have surveyed this mutation in nearly 40 different dog breeds (and mixed-breed dogs) from the United States,[24] Germany,[25] and Brazil (**Fig. 3**).[14] The Irish Wolfhound had the highest allele frequency (42%) followed by the Japanese Beagles (37%–39%) and Berger Blanc Suisse (28%). Interestingly, the beagles studied in Germany[25] and the United States[24] had less than half the allele frequency (15% and 13%, respectively) than the beagles from Japan,[12,13] possibly reflecting colony founder effect differences. The remaining breeds studied had allele frequencies of 10% or less indicating that the likely frequency of the enzyme-deficient homozygous variant dogs would be 1% or less in the population (ie, relatively rare). Interestingly, many of the remaining affected breeds were herding dogs including Australian Shepherd, Collie, Shetland Sheepdog, Bearded Collie, Border Collie, and Old English Sheepdog.[25] Although this could be sampling bias, it might also indicate a common (although

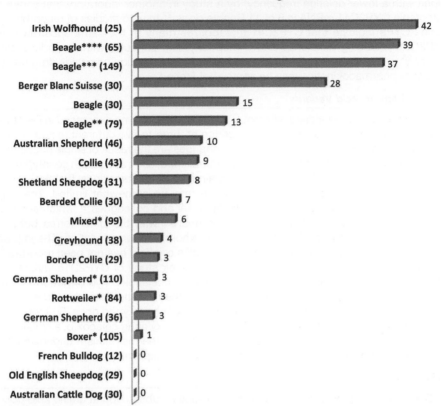

Fig. 3. Allele frequency (number of variant alleles as percent of total alleles) of the CYP1A2 stop codon mutation (R373X) in different dog breeds. Shown after each breed are the numbers of individual dogs that were sampled. Data are from dogs located in Brazil (*Scherr and colleagues[14]); United States (**Whiterock and colleagues[24]); Japan (***Mise and colleagues[13] and ****Tenmisu and colleagues[12]); and Germany (Aretz and Geyer[25]). Only data from breeds in which DNA from at least 10 different dogs in that breed were sampled are shown. Other breeds in which at least one dog had the deficient allele included Whippet, Deerhound, Dalmatian, and Jack Russell Terrier (Aretz and Geyer[25]).

perhaps more recent) ancestry of CYP1A2stop with the MDR1 gene deletion (MDR1del) mutation, which is commonly found in herding breed dogs.[26] The latter results in drug sensitivity from deficiency of the P-glycoprotein transporter encoded by MDR1 (discussed elsewhere in this issue). Regardless, the clinical consequence is that herding breed dogs could be affected by multiple genetic defects (MDR1del and CYP1A2stop) influencing drug disposition and response.

CYP2C41 Gene Deletion

During initial attempts to clone canine CYP2C21 from dog liver RNA, a second CYP2C subfamily enzyme named CYP2C41 was discovered.[16] This latter isoform was found to be present at the RNA and genomic DNA level in only about 16% (4 of 25) of dogs (2 of 10 mixed breeds and 2 of 18 Beagles). This contrasted with CYP2C21 that was found to be expressed in all dogs examined. This finding suggests the presence of a partial or complete deletion of the CYP2C41 gene in many dogs. This was confirmed (albeit with a lower deletion frequency) by a study in another laboratory that showed detectable CYP2C41 mRNA in 6 of 11 Beagle dogs.[27] In vitro studies of recombinant canine CYPs indicate that CYP2C41 metabolizes many of the same substrates as CYP2C21 (including diclofenac and S-mephenytoin), although with much less efficiency.[28,29] Consequently, the impact of the CYP2C41 deletion on canine drug metabolism or pharmacokinetics may be somewhat limited.

CYP2D15 Amino Acid Variants

Several studies have identified different CYP2D15 mRNA forms expressed in liver that vary in predicted amino acid coding sequence at three to five different residues (see **Table 2**). Although it is presumed that these changes are the result of single nucleotide polymorphisms (SNP), this has not yet been established, such as through genotyping of multiple dogs. In vitro studies of expressed amino acid variants suggest that the impact of these coding changes on enzyme function may be somewhat limited. The only exception was the WT2 form identified by Roussel and colleagues,[17] which showed about 50% lower bufuralol hydroxylation compared with the other forms but unchanged celecoxib hydroxylation[18] or dextromethorphan demethylation. The impact of these genetic variants on drug pharmacokinetics or effect has not been reported.

Paulson and colleagues[18] originally undertook their study of CYP2D15 variants to explain polymorphic celecoxib clearance in vivo and celecoxib hydroxylation in vitro in a research colony of Beagle dogs. However, they did not directly address this hypothesis, such as through CYP2D15 genotyping of phenotyped dogs. Furthermore, although CYP2D15 was shown to be capable of hydroxylating celecoxib, a significant role for other CYPs was not excluded. Consequently, the mechanism underlying the celecoxib pharmacokinetic polymorphism remains unexplained.

CYP2E1 Amino Acid Variant

An SNP (1453T>C) resulting in a tyrosine for histidine substitution at amino acid position 485 (H485Y) was discovered during initial cloning of the CYP2E1 cDNA from canine liver RNA.[19] Survey genotyping found an allele frequency of 15% in 100 mixed-breed dogs, and 19% in 13 Beagles. An in vitro study comparing expressed wild-type (485H) and variant (485Y) CYP2E1 isoforms showed no difference in chlorzoxazone hydroxylation activity. However, because only one substrate was evaluated, substrate-dependent effects cannot be excluded. In vivo effects of this SNP on drug pharmacokinetics have not been reported.

CYP3A12 Amino Acid Variants

A variant (called CYP3A12*2) that included five different nucleotide differences from the initial cloned sequence, and predicted to cause five unique amino acid changes, was also discovered during cloning of the CYP3A12 cDNA from canine liver RNA.[18] In vitro experiments showed no effect of these amino acid changes on testosterone 6-β-hydroxylation by recombinant enzymes. Genotype frequencies or any association of genotype with drug metabolism phenotype measured in vivo have not been reported.

OTHER DOG CYPS ASSOCIATED WITH PHENOTYPIC VARIABILITY
CYP2B11 and Breed-related Anesthetic Drug Hypersensitivity

Severely delayed recovery has been reported for certain dog breeds (primarily Greyhounds and possibly other sighthounds) after use of injectable anesthetic agents,

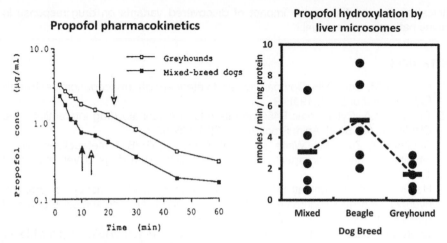

Fig. 4. Greyhounds show slower clearance (*left*) and lower liver metabolism (*right*) of propofol compared with mixed-breed and Beagle dogs. (*Left*) Mean propofol concentrations in 10 Greyhounds and 10 mixed-breed dogs given propofol intravenously at a dose of 5 mg/kg body weight. Time of return of the righting reflex (*solid arrow*) and ability to stand (*open arrow*). (*Right*) Propofol hydroxylation rates measured by high-performance liquid chromatography with in vitro incubations of liver microsomes prepared from male Greyhounds, Beagles, and mixed-breed dogs (five each). The *circles* represent data from individual dog livers. The *horizontal lines* indicate the mean values of each group. ([*Left panel*] *Data from* Zoran DL, Riedesel DH, Dyer DC. Pharmacokinetics of propofol in mixed-breed dogs and greyhounds. Am J Vet Res 1993;54(5):755; [*Right panel*] *Data from* Court MH, Hay-Kraus BL, Hill DW, et al. Propofol hydroxylation by dog liver microsomes: assay development and dog breed differences. Drug Metab Dispos 1999;27(11):1293.)

including thiopental and thiamylal.[30–33] Although initially attributed to decreased drug redistribution from the central compartment resulting from reduced body fat in Greyhounds, a series of studies demonstrated that the effect could be attributed to decreased drug clearance in Greyhounds compared with mixed-breed dogs, and was also prevented by pretreatment with a microsomal enzyme inducer (phenobarbital).[30,31] A subsequent study showed that propofol (another short-acting anesthetic) was also cleared more slowly in Greyhounds,[34] and pretreatment with chloramphenicol, a CYP inhibitor, decreased drug clearance even further (**Fig. 4**).[35] In vitro mechanistic studies identified CYP2B11 as being the main enzyme responsible for CYP-dependent clearance of propofol.[4,36] The molecular genetic basis for this breed-dependent difference in drug metabolism has not been reported.

SUMMARY

Published evidence indicates that variability in drug metabolism by CYP in dogs is likely to be considerable and is explained in part by the presence of genetic polymorphisms that vary between dog breeds. However, few CYPs (mainly CYP1A2) have been systematically investigated, and the influence of the discovered genetic variants on the pharmacokinetics of clinically used drugs and their effects is unclear. Predictions of genetic effects on particular drugs (eg, the effect of CYP1A2 stop codon mutation on phenacetin pharmacokinetics) from human data are complicated by human-dog differences in CYP substrate specificity and abundance. Consequently, clinical studies confirming the impact of discovered variants on drug response in canine patients are essential.

REFERENCES

1. Mosher CM, Court MH. Comparative and veterinary pharmacogenomics. Handb Exp Pharmacol 2010;(199):49.
2. Trepanier LA. Cytochrome P450 and its role in veterinary drug interactions. Vet Clin North Am Small Anim Pract 2006;36(5):975–85, v.
3. Baratta MT, Zaya MJ, White JA, et al. Canine CYP2B11 metabolizes and is inhibited by anesthetic agents often co-administered in dogs. J Vet Pharmacol Ther 2010;33(1):50.
4. Hay Kraus BL, Greenblatt DJ, Venkatakrishnan K, et al. Evidence for propofol hydroxylation by cytochrome P4502B11 in canine liver microsomes: breed and gender differences. Xenobiotica 2000;30(6):575.
5. Court MH, Duan SX, Hesse LM, et al. Cytochrome P-450 2B6 is responsible for interindividual variability of propofol hydroxylation by human liver microsomes. Anesthesiology 2001;94(1):110.
6. Mills BM, Zaya MJ, Walters RR, et al. Current cytochrome P450 phenotyping methods applied to metabolic drug-drug interaction prediction in dogs. Drug Metab Dispos 2010;38(3):396.
7. Zhou D, Linnenbach AJ, Liu R, et al. Expression and characterization of dog cytochrome P450 2A13 and 2A25 in baculovirus-infected insect cells. Drug Metab Dispos 2010;38(7):1015–8.
8. Mise M, Hashizume T, Komuro S. Characterization of substrate specificity of dog CYP1A2 using CYP1A2-deficient and wild-type dog liver microsomes. Drug Metab Dispos 2008;36(9):1903–8.
9. Paine MF, Hart HL, Ludington SS, et al. The human intestinal cytochrome P450 "pie". Drug Metab Dispos 2006;34(5):880.
10. Shimada T, Yamazaki H, Mimura M, et al. Interindividual variations in human liver cytochrome P-450 enzymes involved in the oxidation of drugs, carcinogens and toxic chemicals: studies with liver microsomes of 30 Japanese and 30 Caucasians. J Pharmacol Exp Ther 1994;270(1):414–23.
11. Heikkinen AT, Friedlein A, Lamerz J, et al. Mass spectrometry-based quantification of CYP enzymes to establish in vitro/in vivo scaling factors for intestinal and hepatic metabolism in beagle dog. Pharm Res 2012;29(7):1832–42.
12. Tenmizu D, Endo Y, Noguchi K, et al. Identification of the novel canine CYP1A2 1117 C > T SNP causing protein deletion. Xenobiotica 2004;34(9):835–46.
13. Mise M, Yadera S, Matsuda M, et al. Polymorphic expression of CYP1A2 leading to interindividual variability in metabolism of a novel benzodiazepine receptor partial inverse agonist in dogs. Drug Metab Dispos 2004;32(2):240.
14. Scherr MC, Lourenco GJ, Albuquerque DM, et al. Polymorphism of cytochrome P450 A2 (CYP1A2) in pure and mixed breed dogs. J Vet Pharmacol Ther 2011;34(2):184–6.
15. Whiterock VJ, Morgan DG, Lentz KA, et al. Phenacetin pharmacokinetics in CYP1A2-deficient beagle dogs. Drug Metab Dispos 2012;40(2):228–31.
16. Blaisdell J, Goldstein JA, Bai SA. Isolation of a new canine cytochrome P450 CDNA from the cytochrome P450 2C subfamily (CYP2C41) and evidence for polymorphic differences in its expression. Drug Metab Dispos 1998;26(3):278–83.

17. Roussel F, Duignan DB, Lawton MP, et al. Expression and characterization of canine cytochrome P450 2D15. Arch Biochem Biophys 1998;357(1):27–36.
18. Paulson SK, Engel L, Reitz B, et al. Evidence for polymorphism in the canine metabolism of the cyclooxygenase 2 inhibitor, celecoxib. Drug Metab Dispos 1999;27(10):1133.
19. Lankford SM, Bai SA, Goldstein JA. Cloning of canine cytochrome P450 2E1 cDNA: identification and characterization of two variant alleles. Drug Metab Dispos 2000;28(8):981–6.
20. Tenmizu D, Noguchi K, Kamimura H. Elucidation of the effects of the CYP1A2 deficiency polymorphism in the metabolism of 4-cyclohexyl-1-ethyl-7-methylpyrido 2,3-d pyrimidine-2-(1h)-one (YM-64227), a phosphodiesterase type 4 inhibitor, and its metabolites in dogs. Drug Metab Dispos 2006;34(11):1811.
21. Tenmizu D, Noguchi K, Kamimura H, et al. The canine CYP1A2 deficiency polymorphism dramatically affects the pharmacokinetics of 4-cyclohexyl-1-ethyl-7-methylpyrido 2,3-D -pyrimidine-2-(1H)-one (YM-64227), a phosphodiesterase type 4 inhibitor. Drug Metab Dispos 2006;34(5):800.
22. Azuma R, Komuro M, Kawaguchi Y, et al. Comparative analysis of in vitro and in vivo pharmacokinetic parameters related to individual variability of GTS-21 in canine. Drug Metab Pharmacokinet 2002;17(1):75–82.
23. Kamimura H. Genetic polymorphism of cytochrome P450s in beagles: possible influence of CYP1A2 deficiency on toxicological evaluations. Arch Toxicol 2006; 80(11):732–8.
24. Whiterock VJ, Delmonte TA, Hui LE, et al. Frequency of CYP1A2 polymorphism in beagle dogs. Drug Metab Lett 2007;1(2):163–5.
25. Aretz JS, Geyer J. Detection of the CYP1A2 1117C>T polymorphism in 14 dog breeds. J Vet Pharmacol Ther 2011;34(1):98–100.
26. Neff MW, Robertson KR, Wong AK, et al. Breed distribution and history of canine mdr1-1Delta, a pharmacogenetic mutation that marks the emergence of breeds from the collie lineage. Proc Natl Acad Sci U S A 2004;101(32): 11725.
27. Graham MJ, Bell AR, Crewe HK, et al. mRNA and protein expression of dog liver cytochromes P450 in relation to the metabolism of human CYP2C substrates. Xenobiotica 2003;33(3):225–37.
28. Locuson CW, Ethell BT, Voice M, et al. Evaluation of Escherichia coli membrane preparations of canine CYP1A1, 2B11, 2C21, 2C41, 2D15, 3A12, and 3A26 with coexpressed canine cytochrome P450 reductase. Drug Metab Dispos 2009;37(3):457–61.
29. Shou M, Norcross R, Sandig G, et al. Substrate specificity and kinetic properties of seven heterologously expressed dog cytochromes p450. Drug Metab Dispos 2003;31(9):1161–9.
30. Sams RA, Muir WW. Effects of phenobarbital on thiopental pharmacokinetics in greyhounds. Am J Vet Res 1988;49(2):245.
31. Sams RA, Muir WW, Detra RL, et al. Comparative pharmacokinetics and anesthetic effects of methohexital, pentobarbital, thiamylal, and thiopental in Greyhound dogs and non-Greyhound, mixed-breed dogs. Am J Vet Res 1985; 46(8):1677.
32. Robinson EP, Sams RA, Muir WW. Barbiturate anesthesia in greyhound and mixed-breed dogs: comparative cardiopulmonary effects, anesthetic effects, and recovery rates. Am J Vet Res 1986;47(10):2105.
33. Court MH. Anesthesia of the sighthound. Clin Tech Small Anim Pract 1999; 14(1):38.

34. Zoran DL, Riedesel DH, Dyer DC. Pharmacokinetics of propofol in mixed-breed dogs and greyhounds. Am J Vet Res 1993;54(5):755.
35. Mandsager RE, Clarke CR, Shawley RV, et al. Effects of chloramphenicol on infusion pharmacokinetics of propofol in greyhounds. Am J Vet Res 1995;56(1):95.
36. Court MH, Hay-Kraus BL, Hill DW, et al. Propofol hydroxylation by dog liver microsomes: assay development and dog breed differences. Drug Metab Dispos 1999;27(11):1293.

Feline Drug Metabolism and Disposition
Pharmacokinetic Evidence for Species Differences and Molecular Mechanisms

Michael H. Court, BVSc, PhD

KEYWORDS

- Cat • Species differences • Glucuronidation • Pharmacokinetics

KEY POINTS

- Acetaminophen, propofol, carprofen, and aspirin are eliminated more slowly in cats, and are all metabolized by conjugation.
- Cats lack uridine diphosphate glucuronosyltransferase (UGT) 1A6 and UGT1A9, which glucuronidate acetaminophen and propofol, respectively.
- Slower aspirin clearance results mainly from deficient glycine conjugation and not deficient glucuronidation.
- Cats lack N-acetyltransferase 2, which may be the reason they are prone to developing methemoglobinemia rather than hepatotoxicity from acetaminophen.
- Cats have low thiopurine methyltransferase activity, which causes sensitivity to azathioprine toxicity.
- Piroxicam is eliminated more quickly in cats than in humans and dogs, but the reason for this is unknown.

INTRODUCTION

Veterinarians are well aware that cats are not simply small dogs with regard to their physiology and pharmacology. However, there are few articles that have critically evaluated the evidence for such species differences and their resultant impact on drug efficacy and toxicity in cats. In this article, the primary literature is reviewed, focusing on the available evidence for differences in drug metabolism and disposition between cats, dogs, and humans, as well as the molecular and genetic mechanisms that may explain these differences.

Disclosures: This work was supported by funds provided by the William R. Jones Endowed Chair in Veterinary Medicine at Washington State University. There are no conflicts of interest to report.
Department of Veterinary Clinical Sciences, College of Veterinary Medicine, Washington State University, 100 Grimes Way, Pullman, WA 99164, USA
E-mail address: Michael.Court@vetmed.wsu.edu

Vet Clin Small Anim 43 (2013) 1039–1054
http://dx.doi.org/10.1016/j.cvsm.2013.05.002

DRUG PHARMACOKINETIC DIFFERENCES BETWEEN CATS, DOGS, AND HUMANS

Fig. 1 shows the results of a preliminary survey of the current literature comparing elimination half-life values for 25 different drugs in cats, dogs, and humans. The drugs were chosen to represent a variety of drug elimination mechanisms, including conjugation (n = 8), oxidation (n = 9), and excretion of unchanged drug into the urine and/or bile (n = 8).

Several trends are apparent in **Fig. 1**:

- All of the drugs that are eliminated more slowly in cats (ie, aspirin, propofol, acetaminophen, and carprofen) are cleared by metabolic conjugation, including glucuronidation, sulfation, and/or glycination.
- Piroxicam, which is metabolized mainly by oxidation, is eliminated more rapidly in cats compared with dogs and humans (ie, the opposite of the conjugated drugs).
- Elimination half-life values were highly correlated between dogs and cats for the nonmetabolized drugs, and poorly correlated for the metabolized (oxidized and/or conjugated) drugs.
- Human elimination half-life data were poorly predictive of dog and cat elimination half-life data for most of the drugs evaluated.

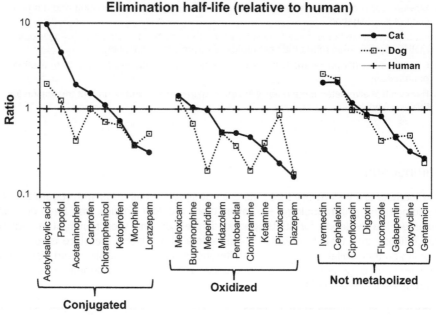

Fig. 1. Pharmacokinetic evidence for differences in drug elimination rates between cats, dogs, and humans. Shown is a comparison of published elimination half-life values in cats (*filled circles*), dogs (*open squares*), and humans (*plus symbols*) for representative drugs that are primarily eliminated by conjugation (glucuronidation, sulfation, and glycination) or oxidation (cytochrome P450 [CYP] enzymes), or that are excreted primarily unchanged into urine and/or bile. All values are expressed as a ratio of the human value. Complete pharmacokinetic data and literature references are given in **Table 1** for acetylsalicylic acid, propofol, acetaminophen, carprofen, and piroxicam. Because of space limitations, the references giving data for other drugs are available directly from the author.

Table 1 lists the elimination half-life, plasma clearance (CL), and volume of distribution (V_d) values of those drugs from **Fig. 1** that had longer (n = 4) or shorter (n = 1) elimination half-life values in cats compared with dogs and humans. The likely mechanisms for these species differences and their implications for drug use in the cat are discussed later.

Acetylsalicylic Acid (Aspirin) and Salicylates

Aspirin is used in cats for acute pain and inflammation or more chronically as an antithrombotic. However, because of slow elimination of aspirin relative to dogs, the recommended doses are 2 to 4 times lower and the dose frequencies are 4 to 6 times longer in cats.[16] Although slow elimination of aspirin in cats has frequently been attributed to deficient glucuronidation,[16] a review of the available literature on aspirin metabolism suggests that other causes are more likely responsible.

After ingestion, aspirin is normally rapidly converted to the major circulating active metabolite, salicylic acid. Salicylic acid is then excreted in the urine unchanged, or following conjugation with glucuronic acid (forming phenolic and acyl glucuronides) or with glycine (forming salicylurate).[17] However, as shown in **Fig. 2**, there is considerable variation in use of these pathways between species. After a therapeutic dose of aspirin (650 mg orally), humans excrete primarily salicylurate (69%), and salicylurate glucuronide (10%), with some salicyl glucuronides (12%) and unchanged salicylate (8%).[17] In comparison, dogs excrete approximately equal amounts of unchanged salicylate, salicylurate, and salicyl glucuronides into their urine after administration of a

Table 1
Pharmacokinetic parameters determined for drugs that have longer (or shorter) elimination half-life values in cats versus dogs and humans. Results are the averages of published studies as referenced. The data from Obach and colleagues[1] (2008), represent a compilation of all available human data up to 2008. Intravenous administration data were used if available to exclude bioavailability differences

Drug	Species	Half-life (h)	CL (mL/min/kg)	V_d (L/kg)
Acetylsalicylic acid[a]	Cat	22	0.088	0.17
	Dog	4.5	0.68	0.29
	Human	2.3	0.66	0.19
Acetaminophen	Cat[b]	5.0	2.9	1.3
	Dog[b]	1.1	13	1.3
	Human[b]	2.6	5	1.0
Propofol	Cat	8.8	17	6.8
	Dog	2.4	51	5.1
	Human	1.9	30	4.7
Carprofen	Cat	18	0.10	0.15
	Dog	12	0.28	0.17
	Human[b]	12	0.48	0.48
Piroxicam	Cat	11	0.52	0.48
	Dog	40	0.044	0.29
	Human[b]	47	0.050	0.16

Abbreviations: CL, plasma clearance; F, bioavailability; V_d, volume of distribution.
[a] Data for disposition of the active metabolite, salicylic acid.
[b] Oral dosing data provided because intravenous or other parental administration data are not available. CL is therefore CL/F and V_d is V_d/F. However, bioavailability for these drugs is considered to be high.
Data from Refs.[1–15]

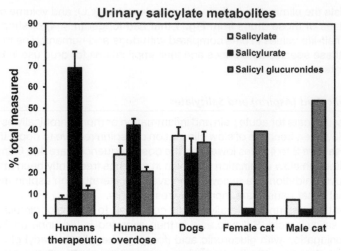

Fig. 2. Cats can readily glucuronidate salicylate, but they poorly conjugate salicylate with glycine (forming salicylurate). Shown are data from several studies comparing the urinary metabolites of salicylate when administered as the sodium salt to 7 dogs and 2 cats (1 male, 1 female) at 44 mg/kg intravenously, or orally as acetylsalicylic acid to 25 human volunteers at a therapeutic dose of 650 mg, or to 24 human patients who had intentionally taken a moderate aspirin overdose. (*Data from* Refs[17,18] and Patel DK, Hesse A, Ogunbona A, et al. Metabolism of aspirin after therapeutic and toxic doses. Hum Exp Toxicol 1990;9(3):131–6.)

44 mg/kg intravenous (IV)dose of sodium salicylate.[18] In the same study, cats excreted mostly salicyl glucuronides (60%–80%) with some unchanged salicylate (12%–23%) but only a minor amount of salicylurate (~5%).

These data suggest that cats can readily glucuronidate salicylic acid, although the type of glucuronide formed is unclear (phenolic and acyl glucuronides are possible). This possibility is supported by in vitro studies that showed significant glucuronidation of salicylic acid by liver tissue slices from cats.[19]

In contrast, the urinary metabolite data (see **Fig. 2**) indicate that cats are deficient in the conjugation of salicylate with glycine to form salicylurate.[18] Although little is known about the enzyme process that mediates salicylic acid glycination, available evidence suggests that it is a 2-step process involving activation of salicylic acid with coenzyme A (Co-A) to form a salicyl-CoA thioester, followed by conjugation with the amino group of glycine to form an amide-linked glycine conjugate.[20] Enzymes thought to be involved in this process in humans include acyl-CoA synthetase medium-chain 2B (ACSM2B, also called HXM-A),[21] and glycine N-acyltransferase (hGLYAT),[22] respectively. Both enzymes are localized to the mitochondrial matrix of liver and kidney tissues. A complementary DNA encoding a feline ortholog of hGLYAT was recently identified (GenBank accession number JV729374),[23] whereas a feline ACSM2B ortholog has yet to be reported.

Slower elimination in cats might be expected for salicylate drugs other than sodium salicylate and aspirin, such as methylsalicylate (oil of wintergreen; Bengay) and trolamine salicylate (Aspercreme), although there is no direct evidence for this in the literature.

Acetaminophen

Although acetaminophen is one of the most widely used nonprescription treatments for mild pain and fever in humans, this drug is rarely used in dogs, and is contraindicated for use in cats. One of the reasons is that dogs, and especially cats, show significant methemoglobinemia and other signs of oxidative injury to erythrocytes (Heinz bodies and anemia) following acetaminophen doses that would be considered nontoxic to humans and other species.[5,24]

In humans, acetaminophen toxicity with increasing doses is typically manifested as acute hepatocellular injury that can proceed to liver failure if not appropriately treated.[25] The mechanism of acetaminophen hepatotoxicity is a consequence of saturation of the major conjugative metabolic pathways (glucuronidation and sulfation) and increased metabolism of acetaminophen by cytochrome P450 (CYP) in liver to form a highly reactive metabolite N-acetyl-p-quinone-imine (NAPQI) (**Fig. 3**).[26] NAPQI is normally detoxified by glutathione conjugation, but once glutathione supplies are depleted (following overdose), NAPQI causes cellular damage. Acetaminophen hepatotoxicity is normally treated by administering the glutathione precursor N-acetylcysteine.

Several explanations for acetaminophen sensitivity in cats have been proposed, including their hemoglobin, which may be more sensitive to oxidative injury, as well as a lower antioxidant capacity of their erythrocytes.[27] However, these explanations do not account for the sensitivity of dogs to methemoglobinemia. Also, NAPQI

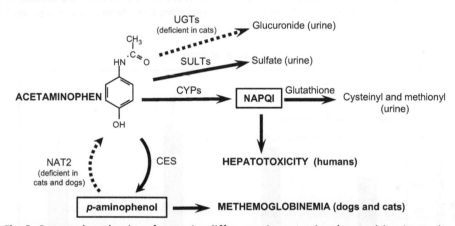

Fig. 3. Proposed mechanisms for species differences in acetaminophen toxicity. Acetaminophen overdose in humans (and most other species) results in acute hepatotoxicity. The mechanism involves saturation of the detoxifying conjugation pathways (sulfation, glucuronidation, and glutathione conjugation), resulting in accumulation of the oxidative reactive metabolite NAPQI in the liver with resultant cellular damage. However, in cats and dogs, acetaminophen toxicity primarily manifests as methemoglobinemia with Heinz body anemia. McConkey and colleagues[27] (2009) proposed the existence of a futile cycle in erythrocytes that involves deacetylation of acetaminophen to p-aminophenol by carboxyesterases (CES) and then reacetylation of p-aminophenol back to acetaminophen by N-acetyltransferase (NAT) isoform 2. p-Aminophenol is a reactive compound that can co-oxidize with hemoglobin to form methemoglobin. Although methemoglobin can be reduced back to hemoglobin by nicotinamide adenine dinucleotide, reduced form, cytochrome b5 reductase, this capacity is limited. p-Aminophenol is proposed to accumulate in cat and dog erythrocytes (and not in humans erythrocytes) because both cat and dog (unlike humans and most other species) lack NAT2. Cats may be more susceptible than dogs to this toxicity because they also lack several uridine diphosphate glucuronosyltransferases (UGTs), including UGT1A6 and UGT1A9, which are essential for efficient elimination of acetaminophen by glucuronidation. Acetaminophen clearance is lower in cats, resulting in increased levels of acetaminophen (and probably p-aminophenol).

is formed by CYPs primarily in the liver and not in the blood. Given the reactivity of this compound, it is unlikely that NAPQI could reach significant levels in erythrocytes. An alternate hypothesis has been explored by McConkey and colleagues[27] (2009), as shown in **Fig. 3**. They propose the existence of a futile cycle in erythrocytes that involves deacetylation of acetaminophen to *p*-aminophenol by carboxyesterases (CES) and then reacetylation of *p*-aminophenol back to acetaminophen by *N*-acetyltransferase (NAT) isoform 2. *p*-Aminophenol is known to be a reactive compound that can co-oxidize with hemoglobin to form methemoglobin. Although methemoglobin can be reduced back to hemoglobin by nicotinamide adenine dinucleotide, reduced form, cytochrome b5 reductase, this capacity is limited. *p*-Aminophenol is proposed to accumulate in cat and dog erythrocytes (and not in human erythrocytes) because both cat and dog (unlike humans and most other species) lack NAT2.

Cats may be more susceptible than dogs to acetaminophen toxicity because they also lack several uridine diphosphate glucuronosyltransferases (UGTs), including UGT1A6 and UGT1A9, which are essential for efficient elimination of acetaminophen by glucuronidation (discussed further later).[28] In support of this, acetaminophen glucuronidation by cat liver microsomes is slow[29] and acetaminophen glucuronide is a minor metabolite of acetaminophen in cat urine, whereas it is the main metabolite in dogs and humans (**Fig. 4**).[5,30,31] As a result, acetaminophen clearance is lower, and

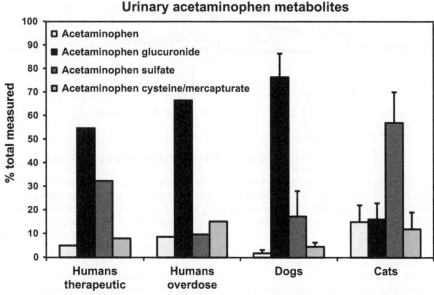

Fig. 4. Cats are sensitive to the toxic effects of acetaminophen, in part because they glucuronidate acetaminophen less efficiently than humans or dogs. Shown are data from several studies comparing the urinary metabolite profiles of acetaminophen following oral administration of a nontoxic dose of 100 mg/kg to 4 dogs, a toxic dose of 120 mg/kg to 6 cats, a therapeutic dose of 20 mg/kg to healthy human volunteers, and an intentional overdose taken by human patients. (*Data from* Savides MC, Oehme FW, Nash SL, et al. The toxicity and biotransformation of single doses of acetaminophen in dogs and cats. Toxicol Appl Pharmacol 1984;74(1):26–34, for cat and dog; and Prescott LF. Kinetics and metabolism of paracetamol and phenacetin. Br J Clin Pharmacol 1980;10 Suppl 2:291S–8S, for human volunteers and overdose patients.)

half-life is longer, in cats (see **Table 1**), resulting in increased circulating levels of acetaminophen, and probably higher p-aminophenol levels in blood.

Propofol

Propofol administered intravenously is commonly used for induction and short-duration anesthesia in dogs and humans. However, repeated dosing or the use of continuous infusions of propofol in cats has been associated with prolonged anesthetic recoveries.[32,33] Furthermore, repeated daily dosing of propofol results in oxidative injury to erythrocytes and increased Heinz body formation after 3 days, and more severe symptoms including malaise, anorexia, and diarrhea after 5 days.[34] A recent study suggested that increasing the dosing interval to 48 hours may ameliorate the more severe symptoms, although there was still evidence for significant Heinz body formation following the first dose.[32]

A toxicity syndrome (called propofol infusion syndrome [PRIS]) in human patients has been associated with administration of high doses of propofol by infusion for up to 48 hours in the intensive care setting.[35,36] The most frequent symptoms include metabolic acidosis, bradyarrhythmias, and progressive myocardial failure, with less frequent symptoms of rhabdomyolysis and renal failure. The mortality is about 80% in published cases, and 30% in cases reported directly to the US Food and Drug Administration. A recent study suggests that the incidence of PRIS is about 1.1% in patients admitted to an intensive care unit and receiving propofol for at least 24 hours, with an 18% mortality.[35] The molecular mechanism underlying PRIS is currently unknown, although various studies have implicated inhibition of several mitochondrial proteins including carnitine palmitoyl-transferase I and the mitochondrial respiratory chain at complex II and IV, either directly by propofol, or by one of its metabolites.[36] It is unknown whether interindividual differences in the metabolism of propofol can contribute to this syndrome.

Propofol is normally eliminated either by glucuronidation (directly) or by CYP-mediated oxidation to form 4-hydroxypropofol that is glucuronidated or sulfated and then excreted into the urine and the bile.[37] The relative use of these pathways differs between species. In humans, about 60% of the dose is eliminated by direct glucuronidation (primarily by UGT1A9), whereas 40% is eliminated by oxidation (primarily by CYP2B6) followed by conjugation.[38,39] However, in dogs, propofol is eliminated almost entirely by oxidation (primarily by CYP2B11) with only 2% of the dose eliminated by direct glucuronidation.[37,40]

However, the metabolism of propofol in cats is unknown. Given that cats do not express an ortholog of UGT1A9,[28] it might be speculated that propofol is mainly metabolized by alternate pathways including oxidation and sulfation. The slow clearance and prolonged elimination half-life of propofol in cats relative to humans and dogs (see **Table 1**) consequently might be explained by deficient glucuronidation in this species. The reason for oxidative injury to feline erythrocytes is less clear, although it might involve the same adverse mitochondrial effects of propofol (or a metabolite) that were proposed as the cause of PRIS in humans. In contrast, propofol is considered to have direct antioxidant effects and has been shown to protect against hemoglobin oxidation, although the antioxidant (or pro-oxidant) effects of its metabolites are unknown.[41]

Carprofen

Carprofen is a nonsteroidal antiinflammatory drug that is commonly used for the treatment of mild to moderate acute and chronic pain in dogs. It is currently approved for use in cats by regulatory agencies in several countries (not the United States) for postoperative analgesia given as a single dose of 4 mg/kg by injection.[42,43] Although longer term use is discouraged because of a lack of safety data, it is also being used orally in cats for treatment of chronic pain.[42] Carprofen was marketed for about 10 years for use in humans, but was withdrawn in 1995 for commercial reasons. The most common adverse side effects are gastrointestinal irritation and ulceration, which are more likely with prolonged use of the oral preparation. Available pharmaco-kinetic data (see **Table 1**) indicate that carprofen is cleared significantly more slowly in cats than in dogs and humans (by 2.8-fold to 4.8-fold) and has a 50% longer half-life. Lower doses and/or a longer dose interval consequently would likely need to be used in cats for chronic administration to achieve the same plasma drug levels as in dogs and humans.

Carprofen is cleared primarily by glucuronidation in the liver.[44] No studies have been published that identify which human UGT glucuronidates carprofen. Slower elimina-tion of carprofen in cats could be a consequence of deficient glucuronidation, although there is no direct evidence to support this. For example, it is not known whether cat liver microsomes glucuronidate carprofen more slowly than human or dog liver. Arguing against this contention is that several structurally related com-pounds, including pirprofen, flurbiprofen, and ibuprofen, are readily glucuronidated by cat liver microsomes.[45] Carprofen is also highly bound to plasma proteins (<1% un-bound in humans and dogs) and so pharmacokinetic differences might also be a consequence of species differences in protein binding, although such an analysis has not been reported.

Piroxicam

Piroxicam is a nonsteroidal antiinflammatory drug that was initially approved for use in humans as an antiinflammatory and analgesic, but has garnered a novel off-label use as a cancer chemotherapeutic in both human and veterinary medicine.[13] Piroxicam pharmacokinetics are different in cats compared with dogs and humans (see **Table 1**). Relative to dogs and humans, cats show more than 10-fold higher clearance of piroxicam and a 3-fold to 4-fold faster elimination half-life. The mechanism for this difference is unclear.

In humans, about 50% of the dose is oxidized by CYP2C9 to 5'-hydroxypiroxicam[46] and most of the remainder is hydrolyzed at the amide bond, presumably by an esterase. Resultant metabolites and some unchanged drug are excreted into urine and bile. 5'-Hydroxypiroxicam is also glucuronidated and excreted in the urine.[47] There is no evidence for direct glucuronidation of piroxicam. Piroxicam (or possibly a metabolite) undergoes significant enterohepatic recirculation in people because pharmacokinetic studies have consistently shown secondary elimination peaks after administration, and a decrease in elimination half-life and faster clearance was observed in people coadministered the anionic sequestrant cholestyramine.[15,48] Pir-oxicam is also highly bound (>99%) to human plasma proteins.[49]

The excretory pathways in dogs are similar to those in humans except that an addi-tional cyclodehydrated metabolite was identified representing as much as 12% of me-tabolites. Pharmacokinetic studies showing strong secondary elimination peaks also suggest that piroxicam undergoes significant enterohepatic recirculation in dogs.[14] The metabolism and excretion of piroxicam in cats is unknown.

Several possibilities exist that might explain faster clearance of piroxicam in cats. Pharmacokinetic elimination profiles of piroxicam in cats do not show any evidence for enterohepatic recirculation (no secondary peaks).[13] As a result, it is possible that the mechanism enabling recirculation in dogs and humans is deficient in cats, leading to faster clearance. An alternative is that cats might have a higher capacity for clearance of piroxicam via hydroxylation or hydrolysis, or by elimination of unchanged drug. In addition, there may be lower plasma protein binding of piroxicam (and/or metabolites) in cats compared with dogs and humans that would tend to favor faster elimination.

MOLECULAR BASIS FOR DIFFERENCES IN CATS VERSUS OTHER SPECIES

Although an understudied area of research, over the last 20 years there has been considerable progress in understanding the molecular and genetic basis for differences in drug metabolism and disposition in cats compared with other species. Deficiencies in 4 different drug elimination pathways have been explored in detail, including glucuronidation (UGTs), acetylation (NATs), methylation (thiopurine methyltransferase [TPMT]), and active transport (ATP-binding cassette G2 [ABCG2]).

Glucuronidation Deficiency

Glucuronidation catalyzed by the UGT enzymes is an important metabolic process that transfers glucuronic acid to many different drugs, toxins, and endogenous compounds (such as steroids and bilirubin), thereby promoting efficient elimination into urine and/or bile. Humans express 19 different UGT isoforms that are classified based on genetic similarity into 2 families and 3 subfamilies (UGT1A, UGT2A, and UGT2B). UGT1A isoforms are encoded by a single gene that produces 9 different enzymes in humans by differential mRNA splicing (**Fig. 5**).[50] Human UGT2A1 and UGT2A2 are also generated by splicing from a single gene, whereas UGT2A3 and all human UGT2B isoforms are products of separate genes.[50] UGTs are primarily expressed in liver, kidney, and intestinal mucosa, which are the primary sites of drug metabolism.[50]

Deficient glucuronidation is one of the oldest and most widely appreciated pharmacologic idiosyncrasies of cats (perhaps second only to so-called morphine mania). Reports regarding the inability of cats to glucuronidate drugs and toxins originated in the scientific literature nearly 60 years ago.[51] Since then various studies have determined that this deficiency in cats is not generalized to all glucuronidated drugs, but depends on drug structure. The defect seems to mainly affect compounds with a simple planar phenolic structure.[52,53]

Studies of UGT isoform substrate specificity in humans and other species indicate that simple planar phenolic compounds are mainly metabolized by several UGT1A isoforms expressed in liver, particularly UGT1A6 and UGT1A9.[29] Furthermore, it has been shown that feline liver only expresses 2 different UGT1A isoforms, including UGT1A1 and UGT1A2, whereas humans express 5 different UGT1As in liver.[28] UGT1A1 is likely to be conserved amongst species because it is essential for glucuronidating and clearing bilirubin. Although little is known about UGT1A2, it is most related to human UGT1A3 and UGT1A4, which glucuronidate drugs containing carboxylic acid and amines. No UGT1A isoform related to UGT1A6 or UGT1A9 was expressed in cat liver. The same study went on to identify the UGT1A6 gene by DNA sequencing but it contained multiple mutations in all cats.[28] This finding suggests that a functional UGT1A6 gene had been present at one point in cats (or a cat species ancestor), but it had been permanently disabled in this species to form what is commonly called a pseudogene.[28] As shown in **Fig. 5**, this finding was confirmed by the recent sequencing of the feline genome, which found only 2 isoforms (UGT1A1 and UGT1A2) and the UGT1A6 pseudogene. In comparison, based on available genome sequences, dogs express up to 10 different UGT1As, whereas humans express 9 different UGT1As (see **Fig. 5**).

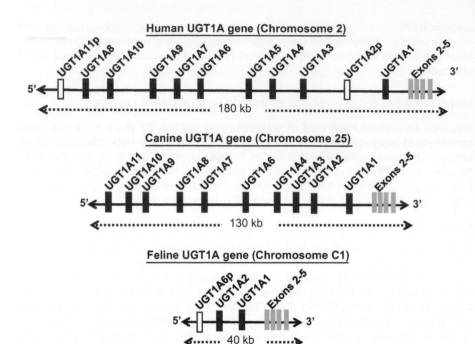

Fig. 5. Comparison of the size, structure, and exon content of the human, canine, and feline UGT1A genes. Each gene consists of multiple exons 1 (designated UGT1A1 to UGT1A11) each with their own promoter that are differentially spliced with the conserved exons 2 to 5. Exon 1 encodes for the UGT enzyme protein domain that binds to and determines substrate specificity, whereas the conserved exons code for the UDPGA-binding domain shared by all UGT1A enzymes. The human gene spans 180 kb and contains 9 functional exons 1 that encode 9 different UGT enzymes. The canine gene is smaller (130 kb) but includes 10 functional exons 1, encoding 10 different UGT enzymes. However, the feline UGT1A gene is smaller (only 40 kb) and has only 2 functional exons 1 that encode 2 different UGT enzymes. Also shown are 2 exons 1 in human and 1 exon 1 in cat that are considered pseudogenes (designated here by the suffix "p" added to the gene name) because they contain multiple mutations that prevent protein coding. UGT1A1 is conserved across all 3 species, probably because it encodes the only known enzyme capable of high-efficiency glucuronidation of bilirubin. (*Data from* Li C, Wu Q. Adaptive evolution of multiple-variable exons and structural diversity of drug-metabolizing enzymes. BMC Evolutionary Biology 2007;7:69 for human and dog genes, and from the University of California at Santa Cruz genome browser for the feline gene.)

Deficient glucuronidation of phenolic compounds has also been shown for other nondomestic felid species, including the African lion and caracal.[54,55] This finding was confirmed by a recent molecular genetic study of a large number of carnivore species that showed UGT1A6 mutations in 17 different nondomestic felid species, representing all major felid lineages, including African lion, tiger, leopard, snow leopard, jaguar, Asiatic golden cat, African golden cat, serval, margay, Geoffrey's cat, tigrina, Canada lynx, bobcat, puma (cougar), Florida panther, cheetah, and leopard cat.[56] However, these mutations in UGT1A6 did not extend beyond the Felidae family to other Carnivora species, such as wolves, ferrets, bears, and raccoons, indicating that the first UGT1A6 mutation had evolved during the separation of the Felidae from other Carnivora species between 11 and 35 million years ago.[56]

In addition, although cats are deficient in several UGT1A enzymes, it is unknown whether other UGT isoforms are also different. In particular, it would be important to know whether cats express feline orthologs of human UGT2B7 and UGT2B15, which glucuronidate many different drugs. UGT2B7 selectively glucuronidates morphine in humans, and there is evidence for reduced morphine glucuronidation by cat liver.[52] This contrasts with the pharmacokinetic data shown in **Fig. 1** indicating that that morphine is eliminated at a similar rate in dogs and even faster than in humans. It is possible that slow morphine glucuronidation in cats may be compensated by clearance through other pathways, including sulfation.[57] UGT2B15 selectively glucuronidates lorazepam in humans, but this benzodiazepine seems to be glucuronidated readily in cats, suggesting that cats express a feline ortholog of human UGT2B15.[58]

Drugs with Evidence for Poor Glucuronidation in Cats

Pharmacology texts and other sources frequently cite deficient glucuronidation as the cause of toxicity or need for dose reduction of glucuronidated drugs given to cats without adequate justification. For example, current evidence points to poor glycine conjugation (discussed earlier) rather than poor glucuronidation as the cause of slow aspirin clearance in cats.[16] **Box 1** lists drugs with clear evidence that they are glucuronidated either more slowly or with similar efficiency compared with other mammalian species. Evidence includes either comparative in vitro glucuronidation studies or in vivo metabolic studies.

Benzyl alcohol and benzoic acid are compounds that are frequently added to drugs as preservatives. Benzyl alcohol is metabolized to benzoic acid and then excreted as the glucuronide or glycine conjugate in most species. Cats are unable to glucuronidate benzoic acid, but can glycinate it, albeit slowly.[63] Benzoic acid poisoning has been reported in cats and it has been recommended that the amounts of benzyl alcohol and benzoic acid used in pharmaceutical preparations for cats be minimized.[64,65]

NAT2 Deficiency

N-Acetylation catalyzed by the N-acetyltransferase enzymes NAT1 and NAT2 is an important metabolic pathway in humans and most other species for several arylamine

---

Box 1
Drugs with direct evidence that they are glucuronidated more slowly (left column) or with similar efficiency (right column) in cats compared with other mammalian species

Drugs glucuronidated slowly in cats	Drugs glucuronidated efficiently in cats
Acetaminophen	Flurbiprofen
Chloramphenicol	Ibuprofen
Clofibrate	Lorazepam
Morphine	Phenolphthalein
Orbifloxacin	Pirprofen
Valproate	Salicylate
	Telmisartan

Data from Refs.[18,29,45,52,53,57–62]

drugs including isoniazid, various sulfonamide antibiotics, dapsone, hydralazine, and procainamide.[66] However, dogs (and all other canid species) lack this metabolic pathway because they lack both genes encoding these enzymes.[67] Cats also lack NAT2, but express NAT1, albeit with lower enzyme activity compared with other species.[66] NAT2 deficiency has been associated with low acetylation of sulfamethazine, sulfanilamide, sulfadimethoxine, and isoniazid by cat liver.[52,66] It is not known whether dapsone and hydralazine are acetylated more slowly in cats. As mentioned earlier, the deficiency of NAT2 in cats, and of both NATs in dogs, are proposed to contribute to the mechanisms of toxicity of acetaminophen that are specific to these species.

TPMT Deficiency

Cats are highly susceptible to the adverse effects of azathioprine.[68] This difference is most likely associated with the low TPMT activity that has been found in cat erythrocytes compared with several other species, including humans.[69–71] S-Methylation by TPMT is an important detoxification mechanism for several drugs used for treatment of cancer (6-mercaptopurine) and for immunosuppression (azathioprine). The reason for the lower TPMT activity in cats is not known but could involve gene sequence differences (from other species) that affect enzyme level and/or enzyme affinity for substrate. Several polymorphisms in the coding sequence of the feline TPMT gene have been identified that affect enzyme protein levels and activity.[69]

ABCG2 Deficiency

Fluoroquinolone antibiotic use has been associated with the development of temporary and permanent blindness in cats.[72] A recent study suggests that this may be the result of inefficient efflux of fluoroquinolones by the ABCG2 transporter from the feline eye.[72] A more complete discussion of this is provided by Mealey elsewhere in this issue.

SUMMARY

Cats are deficient in several drug conjugation pathways that can lead to slow elimination of certain drugs, and the need for dose adjustment or alternative therapies to avoid serious adverse effects. The most well-understood conjugation defect in cats causes reduced glucuronidation of phenolic drugs, such as acetaminophen and propofol. Cats lack UGT1A6 and UGT1A9, which glucuronidate these drugs in other species. Slower clearance of carprofen might also result from deficient glucuronidation, although direct evidence for this is lacking. However, slower aspirin clearance does not seem to result from deficient glucuronidation, and is more likely a consequence of poor glycine conjugation. Cats are also deficient in several other conjugation pathways, including N-acetylation by NAT2 and S-methylation by TPMT. NAT deficiency may be the reason cats (and dogs) are more prone to acetaminophen-induced methemoglobinemia rather than hepatotoxicity. TMPT deficiency likely results in sensitivity to azathioprine toxicity. No evidence was found for slower clearance of drugs that are eliminated by oxidation or unchanged into urine or bile. Piroxicam, an oxidized drug, was cleared more rapidly in cats than in humans and dogs, although the mechanism for this difference is unclear. Species differences in plasma protein binding might also explain observed differences in pharmacokinetics, especially for drugs that are highly bound. Much work is still needed to better understand the molecular causes of drug metabolism and disposition differences in cats, thereby enabling more rational prescribing of existing medications, and the development of more effective and safer drugs for this species.

REFERENCES

1. Obach RS, Lombardo F, Waters NJ. Trend analysis of a database of intravenous pharmacokinetic parameters in humans for 670 drug compounds. Drug Metab Dispos 2008;36(7):1385–405.
2. Parton K, Balmer TV, Boyle J, et al. The pharmacokinetics and effects of intravenously administered carprofen and salicylate on gastrointestinal mucosa and selected biochemical measurements in healthy cats. J Vet Pharmacol Ther 2000;23(2):73–9.
3. Waters DJ, Bowers LD, Cipolle RJ, et al. Plasma salicylate concentrations in immature dogs following aspirin administration: comparison with adult dogs. J Vet Pharmacol Ther 1993;16(3):275–82.
4. Greenblatt DJ, Abernethy DR, Boxenbaum HG, et al. Influence of age, gender, and obesity on salicylate kinetics following single doses of aspirin. Arthritis Rheum 1986;29(8):971–80.
5. Savides MC, Oehme FW, Nash SL, et al. The toxicity and biotransformation of single doses of acetaminophen in dogs and cats. Toxicol Appl Pharmacol 1984;74(1):26–34.
6. Volak LP, Hanley MJ, Masse G, et al. Effect of a herbal extract containing curcumin and piperine on midazolam, flurbiprofen and paracetamol (acetaminophen) pharmacokinetics in healthy volunteers. Br J Clin Pharmacol 2013;75(2):450–62.
7. Cleale RM, Muir WW, Waselau AC, et al. Pharmacokinetic and pharmacodynamic evaluation of propofol administered to cats in a novel, aqueous, nano-droplet formulation or as an oil-in-water macroemulsion. J Vet Pharmacol Ther 2009;32(5):436–45.
8. Lee SH, Ghim JL, Song MH, et al. Pharmacokinetics and pharmacodynamics of a new reformulated microemulsion and the long-chain triglyceride emulsion of propofol in beagle dogs. Br J Pharmacol 2009;158(8):1982–95.
9. Taylor PM, Delatour P, Landoni FM, et al. Pharmacodynamics and enantioselective pharmacokinetics of carprofen in the cat. Res Vet Sci 1996;60(2):144–51.
10. Schmitt M, Guentert TW. Biopharmaceutical evaluation of carprofen following single intravenous, oral, and rectal doses in dogs. Biopharm Drug Dispos 1990;11(7):585–94.
11. Holazo AA, Chen SS, McMahon FG, et al. The influence of liver dysfunction on the pharmacokinetics of carprofen. J Clin Pharmacol 1985;25(2):109–14.
12. Iwakawa S, Suganuma T, Lee SF, et al. Direct determination of diastereomeric carprofen glucuronides in human plasma and urine and preliminary measurements of stereoselective metabolic and renal elimination after oral administration of carprofen in man. Drug Metab Dispos 1989;17(4):414–9.
13. Heeb HL, Chun R, Koch DE, et al. Single dose pharmacokinetics of piroxicam in cats. J Vet Pharmacol Ther 2003;26(4):259–63.
14. Galbraith EA, McKellar QA. Pharmacokinetics and pharmacodynamics of piroxicam in dogs. Vet Rec 1991;128(24):561–5.
15. Guentert TW, Defoin R, Mosberg H. The influence of cholestyramine on the elimination of tenoxicam and piroxicam. Eur J Clin Pharmacol 1988;34(3):283–9.
16. Merck veterinary manual. Available at: http://www.merckvetmanual.com/mvm/index.jsp?cfile=htm/bc/214009.htm. Accessed January 25, 2013.
17. Chen Y, Kuehl GE, Bigler J, et al. UGT1A6 polymorphism and salicylic acid glucuronidation following aspirin. Pharmacogenet Genomics 2007;17(8):571–9.
18. Davis LE, Westfall BA. Species differences in biotransformation and excretion of salicylate. Am J Vet Res 1972;33(6):1253–62.

19. Schachter D, Kass DJ, Lannon TJ. The biosynthesis of salicyl glucuronides by tissue slices of various organs. J Biol Chem 1959;234(1):201–5.
20. Forman WB, Davidson ED, Webster LT Jr. Enzymatic conversion of salicylate to salicylurate. Mol Pharmacol 1971;7(3):247–59.
21. Vessey DA, Lau E, Kelley M, et al. Isolation, sequencing, and expression of a cDNA for the HXM-A form of xenobiotic/medium-chain fatty acid:CoA ligase from human liver mitochondria. J Biochem Mol Toxicol 2003;17(1):1–6.
22. Kelley M, Vessey DA. Isolation and characterization of mitochondrial acyl-CoA: glycine N-acyltransferases from kidney. J Biochem Toxicol 1993;8(2):63–9.
23. Irizarry KJ, Malladi SB, Gao X, et al. Sequencing and comparative genomic analysis of 1227 *Felis catus* cDNA sequences enriched for developmental, clinical and nutritional phenotypes. BMC Genomics 2012;13:31.
24. Nash SL, Savides MC, Oehme FW, et al. The effect of acetaminophen on methemoglobin and blood glutathione parameters in the cat. Toxicology 1984;31(3–4):329–34.
25. Larson AM, Polson J, Fontana RJ, et al. Acetaminophen-induced acute liver failure: results of a United States multicenter, prospective study. Hepatology 2005;42(6):1364.
26. James LP, Mayeux PR, Hinson JA. Acetaminophen-induced hepatotoxicity. Drug Metab Dispos 2003;31(12):1499.
27. McConkey SE, Grant DM, Cribb AE. The role of para-aminophenol in acetaminophen-induced methemoglobinemia in dogs and cats. J Vet Pharmacol Ther 2009;32(6):585–95.
28. Court MH, Greenblatt DJ. Molecular genetic basis for deficient acetaminophen glucuronidation by cats: UGT1A6 is a pseudogene, and evidence for reduced diversity of expressed hepatic UGT1A isoforms. Pharmacogenetics 2000;10(4):355.
29. Court MH, Greenblatt DJ. Molecular basis for deficient acetaminophen glucuronidation in cats. An interspecies comparison of enzyme kinetics in liver microsomes. Biochem Pharmacol 1997;53(7):1041.
30. Gelotte CK, Auiler JF, Lynch JM, et al. Disposition of acetaminophen at 4, 6, and 8 g/day for 3 days in healthy young adults. Clin Pharmacol Ther 2007;81(6):840–8.
31. Prescott LF. Kinetics and metabolism of paracetamol and phenacetin. Br J Clin Pharmacol 1980;10(Suppl 2):291S–8S.
32. Taylor PM, Chengelis CP, Miller WR, et al. Evaluation of propofol containing 2% benzyl alcohol preservative in cats. J Feline Med Surg 2012;14(8):516–26.
33. Pascoe PJ, Ilkiw JE, Frischmeyer KJ. The effect of the duration of propofol administration on recovery from anesthesia in cats. Vet Anaesth Analg 2006;33(1):2–7.
34. Andress JL, Day TK, Day D. The effects of consecutive day propofol anesthesia on feline red blood cells. Vet Surg 1995;24(3):277–82.
35. Roberts RJ, Barletta JF, Fong JJ, et al. Incidence of propofol-related infusion syndrome in critically ill adults: a prospective, multicenter study. Crit Care 2009;13(5):R169.
36. Diedrich DA, Brown DR. Analytic reviews: propofol infusion syndrome in the ICU. J Intensive Care Med 2011;26(2):59–72.
37. Simons PJ, Cockshott ID, Douglas EJ, et al. Species differences in blood profiles, metabolism and excretion of 14C-propofol after intravenous dosing to rat, dog and rabbit. Xenobiotica 1991;21(10):1243–56.

38. Favetta P, Degoute CS, Perdrix JP, et al. Propofol metabolites in man following propofol induction and maintenance. Br J Anaesth 2002;88(5):653–8.
39. Court MH, Duan SX, Hesse LM, et al. Cytochrome P-450 2B6 is responsible for interindividual variability of propofol hydroxylation by human liver microsomes. Anesthesiology 2001;94(1):110.
40. Hay Kraus BL, Greenblatt DJ, Venkatakrishnan K, et al. Evidence for propofol hydroxylation by cytochrome P4502B11 in canine liver microsomes: breed and gender differences. Xenobiotica 2000;30(6):575.
41. Stratford N, Murphy P. Effect of lipid and propofol on oxidation of haemoglobin by reactive oxygen species. Br J Anaesth 1997;78(3):320–2.
42. Lascelles BD, Court MH, Hardie EM, et al. Nonsteroidal anti-inflammatory drugs in cats: a review. Vet Anaesth Analg 2007;34(4):228.
43. Sparkes AH, Heiene R, Lascelles BD, et al. ISFM and AAFP consensus guidelines: long-term use of NSAIDs in cats. J Feline Med Surg 2010;12(7): 521–38.
44. Ray JE, Wade DN. The pharmacokinetics and metabolism of 14C-carprofen in man. Biopharm Drug Dispos 1982;3(1):29–38.
45. Magdalou J, Chajes V, Lafaurie C, et al. Glucuronidation of 2-arylpropionic acids pirprofen, flurbiprofen, and ibuprofen by liver microsomes. Drug Metab Dispos 1990;18(5):692–7.
46. Tracy TS, Hutzler JM, Haining RL, et al. Polymorphic variants (CYP2C9*3 and CYP2C9*5) and the F114L active site mutation of CYP2C9: effect on atypical kinetic metabolism profiles. Drug Metab Dispos 2002;30(4):385–90.
47. Richardson CJ, Blocka KL, Ross SG, et al. Piroxicam and 5'-hydroxypiroxicam kinetics following multiple dose administration of piroxicam. Eur J Clin Pharmacol 1987;32(1):89–91.
48. Hobbs DC, Twomey TM. Piroxicam pharmacokinetics in man: aspirin and antacid interaction studies. J Clin Pharmacol 1979;19(5–6):270–81.
49. Richardson CJ, Blocka KL, Ross SG, et al. Effects of age and sex on piroxicam disposition. Clin Pharmacol Ther 1985;37(1):13–8.
50. Court MH, Zhang X, Ding X, et al. Quantitative distribution of mRNAs encoding the 19 human UDP-glucuronosyltransferase enzymes in 26 adult and 3 fetal tissues. Xenobiotica 2012;42(3):266.
51. Hartiala KJ. Studies on detoxication mechanisms. III. Glucuronide synthesis of various organs with special reference to the detoxifying capacity of the mucous membrane of the alimentary canal. Ann Med Exp Biol Fenn 1955;33(3): 239–45.
52. Gregus Z, Watkins JB, Thompson TN, et al. Hepatic phase I and phase II biotransformations in quail and trout: comparison to other species commonly used in toxicity testing. Toxicol Appl Pharmacol 1983;67(3):430–41.
53. Watkins JB 3rd, Klaassen CD. Xenobiotic biotransformation in livestock: comparison to other species commonly used in toxicity testing. J Anim Sci 1986; 63(3):933–42.
54. French MR, Bababunmi EA, Golding RR, et al. The conjugation of phenol, benzoic acid, 1-naphthylacetic acid and sulphadimethoxine in the lion, civet and genet. FEBS Lett 1974;46(1):134–7.
55. Capel ID, French MR, Millburn P, et al. The fate of (14C)phenol in various species. Xenobiotica 1972;2(1):25–34.
56. Shrestha B, Reed JM, Starks PT, et al. Evolution of a major drug metabolizing enzyme defect in the domestic cat and other Felidae: phylogenetic timing and the role of hypercarnivory. PLoS One 2011;6(3):e18046.

57. Yeh SY, Chernov HI, Woods LA. Metabolism of morphine by cats. J Pharm Sci 1971;60(3):469–71.
58. Schillings RT, Sisenwine SF, Schwartz MH, et al. Lorazepam: glucuronide formation in the cat. Drug Metab Dispos 1975;3(2):85–8.
59. Emudianughe TS, Caldwell J, Sinclair KA, et al. Species differences in the metabolic conjugation of clofibric acid and clofibrate in laboratory animals and man. Drug Metab Dispos 1983;11(2):97–102.
60. Matsumoto S, Takahashi M, Kitadai N, et al. A study of metabolites isolated from the urine samples of cats and dogs administered orbifloxacin. J Vet Med Sci 1998;60(11):1259–61.
61. Zoran DL, Boeckh A, Boothe DM. Hyperactivity and alopecia associated with ingestion of valproic acid in a cat. J Am Vet Med Assoc 2001;218(10):1587–9, 1580.
62. Ebner T, Schanzle G, Weber W, et al. In vitro glucuronidation of the angiotensin II receptor antagonist telmisartan in the cat: a comparison with other species. J Vet Pharmacol Ther 2013;36(2):154–60.
63. Bridges JW, French MR, Smith RL, et al. The fate of benzoic acid in various species. Biochem J 1970;118(1):47–51.
64. Janz R. Benzoic acid hazard in cat preparations. Vet Rec 1989;124(22):595.
65. Bedford PG, Clarke EG. Experimental benzoic acid poisoning in the cat. Vet Rec 1972;90(3):53–8.
66. Trepanier LA, Cribb AE, Spielberg SP, et al. Deficiency of cytosolic arylamine N-acetylation in the domestic cat and wild felids caused by the presence of a single NAT1-like gene. Pharmacogenetics 1998;8(2):169–79.
67. Trepanier LA, Ray K, Winand NJ, et al. Cytosolic arylamine N-acetyltransferase (NAT) deficiency in the dog and other canids due to an absence of NAT genes. Biochem Pharmacol 1997;54(1):73–80.
68. Beale KM, Altman D, Clemmons RR, et al. Systemic toxicosis associated with azathioprine administration in domestic cats. Am J Vet Res 1992;53(7):1236–40.
69. Salavaggione OE, Yang C, Kidd LB, et al. Cat red blood cell thiopurine S-methyltransferase: companion animal pharmacogenetics. J Pharmacol Exp Ther 2004;308(2):617–26.
70. White SD, Rosychuk RA, Outerbridge CA, et al. Thiopurine methyltransferase in red blood cells of dogs, cats, and horses. J Vet Intern Med 2000;14(5):499–502.
71. Foster AP, Shaw SE, Duley JA, et al. Demonstration of thiopurine methyltransferase activity in the erythrocytes of cats. J Vet Intern Med 2000;14(5):552–4.
72. Ramirez CJ, Minch JD, Gay JM, et al. Molecular genetic basis for fluoroquinolone-induced retinal degeneration in cats. Pharmacogenet Genomics 2011;21(2):66–75.

Idiosyncratic Drug Toxicity Affecting the Liver, Skin, and Bone Marrow in Dogs and Cats

Lauren A. Trepanier, DVM, PhD

KEYWORDS

- Adverse drug reaction • Hepatotoxicity • Skin eruption • Blood dyscrasia

KEY POINTS

- Idiosyncratic drug toxicity reactions typically occur in the first 1 to 2 months of drug therapy.
- The presence of a new fever, skin eruption, blood dyscrasia, or hepatopathy (with either a cholestatic or hepatocellular pattern) should raise suspicion for idiosyncratic drug toxicity. Proteinuria, uveitis, arthropathy, or mucocutaneous ulceration can also be seen.
- Management involves early drug discontinuation and, depending on the drug involved, treatment with glutathione precursors, short courses of prednisolone, or intravenous immunoglobulin.

INTRODUCTION

Drug toxicities can be categorized generally as dose dependent or idiosyncratic. For dose-dependent reactions, toxicity increases reliably with dose in one or more species, and most members of a population are affected at high enough dosages. In contrast, idiosyncratic reactions occur in only a small proportion of patients at therapeutic dosages, and are more difficult to predict. Idiosyncratic toxicity does not increase with dose in the general population (therefore they are not considered dose dependent), but toxicity probably does increase with dose in susceptible individuals.

Idiosyncratic drug toxicity is often caused by reactive metabolites, which may be variably generated among individuals (**Fig. 1**). These reactive metabolites typically cause oxidative stress and/or lead to haptens that trigger a humoral or T cell–mediated immunologic response. Although idiosyncratic drug reactions are sometimes called drug hypersensitivity reactions, they may or may not involve an adaptive immune

Disclosures: The author has nothing to disclose.
School of Veterinary Medicine, University of Wisconsin-Madison, 2015 Linden Drive, Madison, WI 53706-1102, USA
E-mail address: latrepanier@svm.vetmed.wisc.edu

Vet Clin Small Anim 43 (2013) 1055–1066
http://dx.doi.org/10.1016/j.cvsm.2013.04.003
0195-5616/13/$ – see front matter © 2013 Elsevier Inc. All rights reserved.

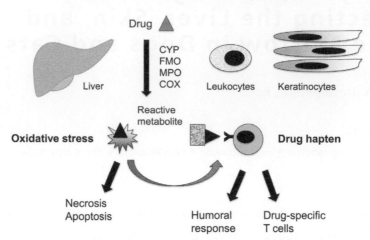

Fig. 1. Most idiosyncratic drug reactions appear to start with a reactive metabolite. These metabolites can be generated by cytochrome P450s (CYP), flavin-monooxygenases (FMO), myeloperoxidases (MPO), or cyclooxygenases (COX). Reactive metabolites or associated reactive oxygen species can cause direct cell or organelle toxicity, or can bind to tissue proteins and form immunogenic haptens. This latter mechanism can lead to amplification of tissue damage through antibody-mediated or T cell–mediated cytotoxicity.

response. Idiosyncratic drug reactions usually require discontinuation of the suspect drug and avoidance of structurally related drugs because they may cause a similar reaction.

TARGETS OF IDIOSYNCRATIC DRUG TOXICITY

The liver, skin, bone marrow, and circulating blood cells are common targets of idiosyncratic drug toxicity. The liver is susceptible because of high blood flow and a high concentration of cytochrome P450s and other biotransformation enzymes that can generate reactive metabolites. Blood cells have a high tissue mass of circulating or dividing cells, which express cytochrome P450s, myeloperoxidases, and cyclooxygenases, each of which can bioactivate certain drugs. In addition, the skin has a large surface area, with a high number of antigen-presenting (Langerhans) cells, and some cytochrome P450 and cyclooxygenase activity in keratinocytes.

DRUGS IMPLICATED IN IDIOSYNCRATIC TOXICITY

This article focuses on the most common drugs associated with idiosyncratic toxicity; less commonly prescribed drugs or those with only single reports of idiosyncratic toxicity are listed in **Table 1**.

Potentiated Sulfonamides

Sulfonamide antibiotics are one of the oldest antimicrobial classes used in veterinary medicine, and are still important for the treatment of methicillin-resistant staphylococcus and fluoroquinolone-resistant gram-negative bacterial infections. However, potentiated sulfonamides can lead to hepatopathy, blood dyscrasias, and skin eruptions, typically after 5 to 14 days of treatment (also known as sulfonamide

Table 1
Other drugs associated with idiosyncratic toxicity in dogs or cats

Drugs in Dogs	Toxicity	Clinical Features, Mechanism(s)	Monitoring and Management
Phenylbutazone	Aplastic anemia in dogs[49]	Oxidation of phenylbutazone to reactive metabolites by blood cell peroxidases[50]	Phenylbutazone not recommended for use in dogs or cats
Fenbendazole	Pancytopenia, bone marrow necrosis in dogs[29,51]	Not established; onset within 2 wk of starting fenbendazole	Very rare; routine monitoring of CBC not indicated
Flucytosine	Skin eruptions with depigmentation and ulceration[52]	Median onset 2–6 wk after starting flucytosine Nasal planum, scrotum, and mucocutaneous junctions affected	Clinical vigilance, drug discontinuation, and supportive care
Mitotane	Hepatopathy (mixed hepatocellular and cholestatic pattern)[53] Bone marrow necrosis[29]	Hepatopathy seen after 1 mo of treatment (single case)[53]	Hepatopathy and bone marrow lesions apparently rare
Griseofulvin	Neutropenia or pancytopenia in cats[54,55] Pancytopenia in a dog[56]	Neutropenia reported in FIV-positive cats; recurrent with rechallenge[55] Toxicity not reproducible in cats given high dosages[57]	Alternatives to griseofulvin recommended
Albendazole	Bone marrow suppression in a cat[58]	One case report, erythroid and megakaryocytic lines affected, mechanism unknown Reported in humans with underlying cirrhosis	Reversible with drug discontinuation and supportive care
Meloxicam	Vasculitis with ulcers, vesicles, and erosions in a dog[30]	Noted within 2 d of starting drug, which is atypical for a drug hypersensitivity reaction with first exposure	Apparently rare

Abbreviations: CBC, complete blood count; FIV, feline immunodeficiency virus.

hypersensitivity). Keratoconjunctivitis sicca may also be seen, but this occurs in about 15% of treated dogs,[1] often after a month or more of administration, and does not fit a classic idiosyncratic pattern, although its pathogenesis is not entirely understood.

Clinical presentation of idiosyncratic sulfonamide toxicity
- Fever (50% of cases)[2]
- Hepatocellular necrosis, cholestasis, or both

- Transient neutropenia
- Thrombocytopenia
- Hemolytic anemia (Coomb negative or positive)
- Skin eruptions
  - Vasculitis
  - Pemphigus foliaceus[3]
  - Bullous skin eruptions (erythema multiforme, Stevens-Johnson syndrome, or toxic epidermal necrolysis)
- Polyarthropathy
- Proteinuria
- Uveitis

Sulfonamide hypersensitivity reactions are caused by an oxidized hydroxylamine metabolite that is generated by cytochrome P450s and myeloperoxidases. This hydroxylamine can circulate in the plasma, and spontaneously oxidizes to a reactive nitroso metabolite that covalently binds to proteins and acts as a hapten.[4] Drug-specific T cells, some of which have been shown to mediate toxicity against keratinocytes, have been found in human patients,[5] and drug-specific T cells may also occur in dogs. In addition, dogs with sulfonamide hypersensitivity develop antidrug antibodies that cross react with sulfamethoxazole, sulfadiazine, and sulfadimethoxine in about 30% of dogs.[6] In dogs with thrombocytopenia following sulfonamide antimicrobials, antiplatelet antibodies are present, which recognize noncovalent drug-platelet complexes.[7] Some of these antibodies require the continuous presence of sulfonamide drug to bind to platelets, which may explain why thrombocytopenia may resolve rapidly in some dogs after sulfonamide discontinuation.

Risk factors for sulfonamide hypersensitivity in dogs are not clear. Brand name and generic formulations have each been implicated.[2] Doberman pinschers seem to be over-represented among dogs with the combination of polyarthropathy, thrombocytopenia, and proteinuria.[8,9] Human patients with sulfonamide hypersensitivity may also cross react with structurally related arylamine drugs such as dapsone[10] and sulfapyridine (found in sulfasalazine).[11] However, there is no clear evidence of cross reactivity between sulfonamide antibiotics and nonarylamine drugs containing a sulfonamide group, such as furosemide, acetazolamide, and hydrochlorthiazide.[12] Despite the term sulfonamide hypersensitivity, it is the arylamine moiety, and not the sulfonamide part of the drug, that is involved in hapten generation.

Management of suspected sulfonamide hypersensitivity
- Owner vigilance for adverse events
- Stop potentiated sulfonamide at first sign of illness
- Supportive care
- Consider treatment with antioxidants:
  - Ascorbate and glutathione decrease binding of sulfonamide metabolites to dog liver proteins in vitro (Lavergne and Trepanier, unpublished data, 2005)
    - Ascorbate 90 mg/kg/d intravenous (IV) (empiric dosage)
    - N-acetylcysteine 140 mg/kg loading IV, then 70 mg/kg every 6 hours for 7 treatments (as for acetaminophen toxicosis)
- Consider short course of prednisone (2–3 months)
  - If persistent thrombocytopenia or hemolytic anemia
- Consider IV immunoglobulin
  - Anecdotal success for sulfonamide-associated bullous skin eruptions in a dog (IV immunoglobulin G at 0.5 g/kg)[13]

Methimazole

In cats, the antithyroid drug methimazole is also associated with idiosyncratic toxicity affecting the liver, skin, and blood cells. Similar reactions have also been reported for carbimazole, which is a prodrug of methimazole (see the carbimazole [Vidalta] label).

Methimazole hepatotoxicity shows a mixed hepatocellular and cholestatic pattern in cats, and typically occurs in the first month of treatment, with a 1% to 2% incidence of jaundice.[14] Drug-induced increases in liver enzymes resolve within several weeks of methimazole discontinuation, although clinical improvement is more rapid. Rechallenge has led to recrudescence of hepatotoxicity.[14] These changes are distinct from innocent increases in alanine aminotransferase (ALT) and serum alkaline phosphatase (SAP) seen in cats with hyperthyroidism, which resolve with a return to the euthyroid state and do not worsen during antithyroid drug treatment.

Methimazole hepatotoxicity also occurs in about 9% of human patients, with a mean onset of 28 days after starting the drug.[15] Hepatotoxicity has been observed in a rodent model, and is associated with an N-methylthiourea metabolite that is generated by flavin monooxygenases.[16,17] Glutathione depletion is an experimental risk factor for methimazole hepatotoxicity,[16] and either N-acetylcysteine or taurine attenuate hepatocyte toxicity in vitro.[18,19] These findings may have relevance for methimazole hepatotoxicity in cats. Although we recently found no association between glutathione depletion and idiosyncratic methimazole toxicity in pet cats,[20] cats were tested after their adverse reactions instead of before methimazole administration, and only blood, not hepatic, glutathione was measured.

Blood dyscrasias are seen in about 4% of cats treated with methimazole, and include thrombocytopenia and neutropenia or agranulocytosis.[14] These reactions typically occur in the first 1 to 2 months of treatment, and rechallenge has led to recurrence. Monitoring for blood dyscrasias is important, because these reactions can progress to bleeding or secondary infections.

In humans, methimazole-induced and carbimazole-induced blood dyscrasias are well described, to include thrombocytopenia, hemolytic anemia, neutropenia, and agranulocytosis. These reactions seem to be immune mediated, but can occur after years of therapy.[21] Drug-dependent antibodies targeting neutrophils (FcγRIIIb) and erythrocytes (Rh complex proteins) have been shown, as well as antibodies that bind to the adhesion molecule PECAM-1 in the presence of drug.[21] PECAM-1 (also known as CD31) is expressed on platelets, neutrophils, and monocytes, and antibodies against this molecule may explain the involvement of multiple cell lineages in these blood dyscrasias. In addition, the requirement of drug for antibody binding in vitro is consistent with the development of transient protein-drug neoantigens. Such a scenario is also consistent with the clinical observation of rapid recovery of cell counts after drug discontinuation in cats, although methimazole-dependent or carbimazole-dependent antibodies in cats have yet to be evaluated.

Pruritus and facial excoriation develops in 2% to 3% of cats treated with methimazole, most commonly in the first 3 weeks of treatment.[14] Lesions are typically caused by self-trauma of the neck and the face anterior to the pinnae, but have not been characterized histologically. Pruritus and urticaria are also seen in about 8% of pediatric patients[22] and up to 20% of adults[15] treated with methimazole, typically in the first 4 weeks of treatment. More severe bullous skin eruptions such as Stevens-Johnson syndrome have also been reported.[22] The mechanisms for these reactions have not been explored.

Prevention and management of methimazole toxicity
- Counsel owners to monitor for lethargy, vomiting, inappetence, jaundice, or pruritus.
- Stop drug at first potential sign of adverse reaction.
- Evaluate cat as soon as possible:
  - Physical examination for skin excoriations
  - Rule out blood dyscrasia (complete blood count [CBC])
  - Rule out hepatotoxicity (ALT, bilirubin, SAP)
    - Compare with pretreatment liver enzymes (often reversibly increased in hyperthyroid cats)
  - Evaluate for renal decompensation (blood urea nitrogen [BUN], creatinine, serum T4)
- If simple gastrointestinal (GI) upset (normal blood work):
  - Plan dose reduction or switch to transdermal methimazole, which has a lower incidence of GI upset than oral methimazole[23]
- If blood dyscrasia, hepatopathy, or facial excoriation:
  - Plan radioiodine, or, if not available, thyroidectomy with atenolol pretreatment
  - The efficacy of glutathione precursors or glucocorticoids has not been evaluated for methimazole in this setting.

Carprofen

Carprofen is commonly thought to have a higher risk of hepatotoxicity than other nonsteroidal antiinflammatory drugs (NSAIDs), but this has not been shown in a comparative study. The veterinary labels for meloxicam, etodolac, deracoxib, firocoxib, and robenacoxib also report liver toxicity in dogs. However, idiosyncratic carprofen hepatotoxicity has been described in the greatest detail.

Clinical presentation of carprofen hepatoxicity[24]
- Most dogs affected within 14 to 30 days
- Acute hepatic necrosis with marked increases in ALT
  - No reported cases of carprofen hepatotoxicity have had increases in SAP without large accompanying increases in ALT[24]
- Labrador retrievers were over-represented in the initial report, but the manufacturer could not reproduce this syndrome in Labrador dogs (personal communication, Dr. Terry Clark, 2002). Therefore, this is unlikely to be a true breed risk.
- Manufacturer's report rate: fewer than 5 cases per 10,000 dogs treated (<0.05%)
  - Hepatic dysfunction in less than 0.02% of treated dogs

Idiosyncratic NSAID hepatotoxicity also occurs in human patients,[25] with diclofenac implicated most commonly. Threefold or higher increases in ALT occur in about 5% of patients, with hepatocellular necrosis in the first 6 months of diclofenac treatment seen much less commonly. Diclofenac metabolites cause mitochondrial injury in vitro,[26] which could explain mild transaminase increases in some patients. The progression to hepatocellular necrosis could involve an amplification of this cytotoxicity by an immune response to drug haptens, in particular those formed by reactive acyl-glucuronide and quinone imine diclofenac metabolites.[27] Carprofen shares some structural similarities with diclofenac, so a similar scenario could apply to carprofen as well. This topic requires further evaluation.

NSAID-associated blood dyscrasias and skin eruptions have been reported in isolated case reports in veterinary patients, to include thrombocytopenia and hemolytic anemia (1 case) and bone marrow necrosis (3 cases) during carprofen treatment,[28,29] and vasculitis during meloxicam or carprofen treatment (1 case each).[28,30]

Although hepatotoxicity, cytopenias, and vasculitis from NSAIDs can be severe, these idiosyncratic reactions are rare, and are not efficiently detected by routine biochemical monitoring. Clinical monitoring by owners is key, and every client should be advised to monitor for new vomiting, diarrhea, lethargy, skin lesions, or change in urine color. Dose-dependent gastric ulceration and new azotemia are more common, and deserve routine clinical monitoring. Middle-aged to older dogs are more likely to have preexisting organ dysfunction, and should have baseline blood work performed to evaluate hematocrit, BUN, creatinine, albumin, and ALT before starting NSAID treatment. Abnormal clinical signs during NSAID treatment in any dog should prompt drug discontinuation; a physical examination, CBC, and biochemical panel can distinguish between simple GI upset, gastric ulceration, renal compensation, or idiosyncratic reactions.

Zonisamide

Acute hepatotoxicity was recently reported in 2 dogs treated with the anticonvulsant drug zonisamide.[31,32] In both dogs, clinical signs developed in the first 3 weeks of treatment, one with a hepatocellular pattern and one with a mixed hepatocellular and cholestatic pattern. Liver failure progressed in 1 dog; necropsy showed massive hepatic necrosis with marked periportal microvesicular steatosis. Further clinical experience is needed before the incidence of zonisamide hepatotoxicity is clear; however, dog owners should be informed of this potential adverse drug reaction when zonisamide is prescribed. Clients should be advised to watch for signs of lethargy, GI upset, change in mucous membrane color, or dark urine.

Diazepam

Oral diazepam has led to idiosyncratic acute hepatic necrosis in some cats.[33,34] Affected cats have been otherwise healthy and treated for behavioral problems or urethrospasm; clinical signs were typically seen after 8 to 9 days of treatment. Both generic and brand name oral diazepam have been implicated, although injectable diazepam has not.[33] The time frame for toxicity suggests an immune component (humoral or T-cell mediated), although this has not been explored. Reactions are fulminant and often fatal, but aggressive supportive care can be successful.[35] Acute idiosyncratic liver injury from benzodiazepines is seen uncommonly in human patients,[36,37] so potential mechanisms have not been explored.

Phenobarbital

Phenobarbital hepatotoxicity typically occurs in dogs after a year or more of phenobarbital treatment, and can present with asymptomatic increases in bile acids, clinical signs of hepatic disease, or overt liver failure.[38] The clinical presentation does not follow a classic idiosyncratic or dose-dependent pattern; it is seen late in the course of treatment, and can resolve with dose reduction; however, it has not been reported with loading doses or been reproduced in experimental studies.[39,40]

Phenobarbital hepatotoxicity is probably best described as dose/duration dependent with individual modifiers, but individual risk factors are not clear. Hepatotoxicity could be related to cytochrome P450 induction by phenobarbital, with secondary bioactivation of dietary or environmental compounds. Primidone and phenytoin, which are also cytochrome P450 inducers, lead to a similar pattern of delayed hepatotoxicity.[41] In contrast, phenobarbital in cats leads to neither cytochrome P450 induction[42,43] nor hepatotoxicity. Given the popularity of phenobarbital as an anticonvulsant in dogs, this adverse reaction deserves further study.

Prevention and management of phenobarbital hepatotoxicity
- Use the minimal effective dosage of phenobarbital; consider combination therapy with bromide or other anticonvulsants.
- Evaluate serum bile acids every 6 months during phenobarbital treatment.
- Monitor for inappetence, vomiting, diarrhea, or increased sedation (which can signal decreased hepatic clearance of phenobarbital).
- Screen liver function tests if clinically ill (albumin, bilirubin, BUN, cholesterol, glucose, bile acids, and coagulation profile).
- If hepatopathy develops, plan phenobarbital discontinuation or substantial dose reduction.
- Consider transitioning to KBr monotherapy (40–60 mg/kg/d).
  - Rapid taper of phenobarbital over 1 to 2 weeks
  - KBr loading dose of 400 to 600 mg/kg if brittle epilepsy and no hepatic encephalopathy

In addition to liver toxicity, phenobarbital has rarely been associated with blood dyscrasias in dogs. Abnormalities have included thrombocytopenia, neutropenia, and anemia, with bone marrow necrosis or myelofibrosis noted on bone marrow evaluation.[29,44,45] These reactions respond to drug discontinuation and supportive care unless advanced myelofibrosis has developed.

In human patients, anticonvulsant hypersensitivity syndrome, which can include thrombocytopenia, leukopenia, anemia, and hepatopathy, has also been associated with phenobarbital, with a different clinical presentation than in dogs. This syndrome typically occurs within the first 3 weeks of starting treatment, with a delay of 6 days or more. Reactions may be accompanied by fever, eosinophilia, lymphadenopathy, and skin eruptions,[46] and share many clinical features with sulfonamide hypersensitivity. Patients are managed with drug discontinuation, along with weeks to months of antiinflammatory to immunosuppressive dosages of glucocorticoids in some cases, and IV immunoglobulin in severely affected patients.[46] If hepatopathy is also present, patients are treated with N-acetylcysteine. These reactions may be caused by reactive arene oxide metabolites that form protein-drug haptens and elicit a secondary immune response. Drug-specific T cells have been shown in human patients with hypersensitivity reactions to anticonvulsants that are structurally related to phenobarbital.[47]

In addition, phenobarbital has been associated with skin lesions in dogs; in particular, superficial necrolytic dermatitis. About 45% of cases of superficial necrolytic dermatitis (also called necrolytic migratory erythema or hepatocutaneous syndrome) in dogs are associated with phenobarbital administration.[48] Skin lesions are characterized by hyperkeratosis, crusting, and erythema of the footpads, mucocutaneous junctions, and nasal planum. These lesions develop only after prolonged treatment (a median of 7 years) and are associated with hepatopathy; therefore, the pattern is not consistent with idiosyncratic drug toxicity. The presentation is distinct from the skin eruptions seen in human patients treated with phenobarbital, which occur early in treatment (within the first 2 months) and are not related to any accompanying liver toxicity.[46]

SUMMARY: MONITORING FOR DRUG-INDUCED IDIOSYNCRATIC TOXICITIES

- Obtain a current drug history at every visit
- Always consider a possible adverse drug reaction in your differential list
  - Higher index of suspicion for an idiosyncratic reaction when clinical signs develop within 4 weeks of starting a new drug

- If clinical signs develop:
  - Evaluate for new 3-fold or higher increases in ALT, or cholestasis with jaundice
  - Screen for regenerative or nonregenerative cytopenias
  - Perform careful examination of skin and mucocutaneous junctions
  - Also evaluate for uveitis, joint effusion, or proteinuria
- When in doubt, discontinue all suspect drugs and reintroduce essential drugs one at a time, with careful clinical and biochemical monitoring after each drug addition. Allow 1 to 2 weeks between each drug addition.

REFERENCES

1. Berger S, Scagliotti R, Lund E. A quantitative study of the effects of Tribrissen on canine tear production. J Am Anim Hosp Assoc 1995;31:236–41.
2. Trepanier L, Danhof R, Toll J, et al. Clinical findings in 40 dogs with hypersensitivity associated with administration of potentiated sulfonamides. J Vet Intern Med 2003;17:647–52.
3. White S, Carlotti D, Pin D, et al. Putative drug-related pemphigus foliaceus in four dogs. Vet Dermatol 2002;13:195–202.
4. Naisbitt D, Gordon S, Pirmohamed M, et al. Antigenicity and immunogenicity of sulphamethoxazole: demonstration of metabolism-dependent haptenation and T-cell proliferation in vivo. Br J Pharmacol 2001;133:295–305.
5. Schnyder B, Frutig K, Mauri-Hellweg D, et al. T-cell-mediated cytotoxicity against keratinocytes in sulfamethoxazol-induced skin reaction. Clin Exp Immunol 1998;28:1412–7.
6. Lavergne SN, Danhof RS, Volkman EM, et al. Association of drug-serum protein adducts and anti-drug antibodies in dogs with sulphonamide hypersensitivity: a naturally occurring model of idiosyncratic drug toxicity. Clin Exp Allergy 2006; 36:907–15.
7. Lavergne SN, Trepanier LA. Anti-platelet antibodies in a natural animal model of sulphonamide-associated thrombocytopaenia. Platelets 2007;18:595–604.
8. Giger U, Werner LL, Millichamp NJ, et al. Sulfadiazine-induced allergy in six Doberman pinschers. J Am Vet Med Assoc 1985;186:479–84.
9. Vasilopulos RJ, Mackin A, Lavergne SN, et al. Nephrotic syndrome associated with administration of sulfadimethoxine/ormetoprim in a dobermann. J Small Anim Pract 2005;46:232–6.
10. Jorde UP, Horowitz HW, Wormser GP. Utility of dapsone for prophylaxis of Pneumocystis carinii pneumonia in trimethoprim-sulfamethoxazole-intolerant, HIV-infected individuals. AIDS 1993;7:355–9.
11. Zawodniak A, Lochmatter P, Beeler A, et al. Cross-reactivity in drug hypersensitivity reactions to sulfasalazine and sulfamethoxazole. Int Arch Allergy Immunol 2010;153:152–6.
12. Strom BL, Schinnar R, Apter AJ, et al. Absence of cross-reactivity between sulfonamide antibiotics and sulfonamide nonantibiotics. N Engl J Med 2003; 349:1628–35.
13. Nuttall TJ, Malham T. Successful intravenous human immunoglobulin treatment of drug-induced Stevens-Johnson syndrome in a dog. J Small Anim Pract 2004; 45:357–61.
14. Peterson ME, Kintzer PP, Hurvitz AI. Methimazole treatment of 262 cats with hyperthyroidism. J Vet Intern Med 1988;2:150–7.
15. Otsuka F, Noh JY, Chino T, et al. Hepatotoxicity and cutaneous reactions after antithyroid drug administration. Clin Endocrinol 2012;77:310–5.

16. Mizutani T, Murakami M, Shirai M, et al. Metabolism-dependent hepatotoxicity of methimazole in mice depleted of glutathione. J Appl Toxicol 1999;19:193–8.

17. Mizutani T, Yoshida K, Murakami M, et al. Evidence for the involvement of N-methylthiourea, a ring cleavage metabolite, in the hepatotoxicity of methimazole in glutathione-depleted mice: structure-toxicity and metabolic studies. Chem Res Toxicol 2000;13:170–6.

18. Heidari R, Babaei H, Ali Eghbal M. Mechanisms of methimazole cytotoxicity in isolated rat hepatocytes. Drug Chem Toxicol 2012. [Epub ahead of print].

19. Heidari R, Babaei H, Eghbal MA. Ameliorative effects of taurine against methimazole-induced cytotoxicity in isolated rat hepatocytes. Sci Pharm 2012; 80:987–99.

20. Branter E, Drescher N, Padilla M, et al. Antioxidant status in hyperthyroid cats before and after radioiodine treatment. J Vet Intern Med 2012;26:582–8.

21. Bux J, Ernst-Schlegel M, Rothe B, et al. Neutropenia and anaemia due to carbimazole-dependent antibodies. Br J Haematol 2000;109:243–7.

22. Rivkees SA, Stephenson K, Dinauer C. Adverse events associated with methimazole therapy of Graves' disease in children. Int J Pediatr Endocrinol 2010; 2010:176970.

23. Sartor LL, Trepanier LA, Kroll MM, et al. Efficacy and safety of transdermal methimazole in the treatment of cats with hyperthyroidism. J Vet Intern Med 2004;18:651–5.

24. MacPhail CM, Lappin MR, Meyer DJ, et al. Hepatocellular toxicosis associated with administration of carprofen in 21 dogs. J Am Vet Med Assoc 1998;212: 1895–901.

25. Rostom A, Goldkind L, Laine L. Nonsteroidal anti-inflammatory drugs and hepatic toxicity: a systematic review of randomized controlled trials in arthritis patients. Clin Gastroenterol Hepatol 2005;3:489–98.

26. O'Connor N, Dargan PI, Jones AL. Hepatocellular damage from non-steroidal anti-inflammatory drugs. QJM 2003;96:787–91.

27. Aithal GP, Day CP. Nonsteroidal anti-inflammatory drug-induced hepatotoxicity. Clin Liver Dis 2007;11:563–75, vi–vii.

28. Mellor PJ, Roulois AJ, Day MJ, et al. Neutrophilic dermatitis and immune-mediated haematological disorders in a dog: suspected adverse reaction to carprofen. J Small Anim Pract 2005;46:237–42.

29. Weiss DJ. Bone marrow necrosis in dogs: 34 cases (1996-2004). J Am Vet Med Assoc 2005;227:263–7.

30. Niza MM, Felix N, Vilela CL, et al. Cutaneous and ocular adverse reactions in a dog following meloxicam administration. Vet Dermatol 2007;18:45–9.

31. Miller ML, Center SA, Randolph JF, et al. Apparent acute idiosyncratic hepatic necrosis associated with zonisamide administration in a dog. J Vet Intern Med 2011;25:1156–60.

32. Schwartz M, Munana KR, Olby NJ. Possible drug-induced hepatopathy in a dog receiving zonisamide monotherapy for treatment of cryptogenic epilepsy. J Vet Med Sci 2011;73(11):1505–8.

33. Center SA, Elston TH, Rowland PH, et al. Fulminant hepatic failure associated with oral administration of diazepam in 11 cats. J Am Vet Med Assoc 1996; 209:618–25.

34. Levy J, Cullen J, Bunch S, et al. Adverse reaction to diazepam in cats. J Am Vet Med Assoc 1994;205:156–7.

35. Park FM. Successful treatment of hepatic failure secondary to diazepam administration in a cat. J Feline Med Surg 2012;14:158–60.

36. Sabate M, Ibanez L, Perez E, et al. Risk of acute liver injury associated with the use of drugs: a multicentre population survey. Aliment Pharmacol Ther 2007;25: 1401–9.
37. Tedesco FJ, Mills LR. Diazepam (Valium) hepatitis. Dig Dis Sci 1982;27:470–2.
38. Dayrell-Hart B, Steinberg SA, VanWinkle TJ, et al. Hepatotoxicity of phenobarbital in dogs: 18 cases (1985-1989). J Am Vet Med Assoc 1991;199:1060–6.
39. Aitken MM, Hall E, Scott L, et al. Liver-related biochemical changes in the serum of dogs being treated with phenobarbitone. Vet Rec 2003;153:13–6.
40. Chauvet AE, Feldman EC, Kass PH. Effects of phenobarbital administration on results of serum biochemical analyses and adrenocortical function tests in epileptic dogs. J Am Vet Med Assoc 1995;207:1305–7.
41. Bunch SE, Baldwin BH, Hornbuckle WE, et al. Compromised hepatic function in dogs treated with anticonvulsant drugs. J Am Vet Med Assoc 1984;184:444–8.
42. Maugras M, Reichart E. The hepatic cytochrome level in the cat (*Felis catus*): normal value and variations in relation to some biological parameters. Comp Biochem Physiol B 1979;64:125–7.
43. Truhaut R, Ferrando R, Graillot C, et al. Induction of cytochrome P 450 by phenobarbital in cats. C R Acad Sci Hebd Seances Acad Sci D 1978;286: 371–3 [in French].
44. Jacobs G, Calvert C, Kaufman A. Neutropenia and thrombocytopenia in three dogs treated with anticonvulsants. J Am Vet Med Assoc 1998;212:681–4.
45. Weiss DJ, Smith SA. A retrospective study of 19 cases of canine myelofibrosis. J Vet Intern Med 2002;16:174–8.
46. Newell BD, Moinfar M, Mancini AJ, et al. Retrospective analysis of 32 pediatric patients with anticonvulsant hypersensitivity syndrome (ACHSS). Pediatr Dermatol 2009;26:536–46.
47. Hanafusa T, Azukizawa H, Matsumura S, et al. The predominant drug-specific T-cell population may switch from cytotoxic T cells to regulatory T cells during the course of anticonvulsant-induced hypersensitivity. J Dermatol Sci 2012;65: 213–9.
48. March PA, Hillier A, Weisbrode SE, et al. Superficial necrolytic dermatitis in 11 dogs with a history of phenobarbital administration (1995-2002). J Vet Intern Med 2004;18:65–74.
49. Weiss DJ, Klausner JS. Drug-associated aplastic anemia in dogs: eight cases (1984-1988). J Am Vet Med Assoc 1990;196:472–5.
50. Uetrecht J. Drug metabolism by leukocytes and its role in drug-induced lupus and other idiosyncratic drug reactions. Crit Rev Toxicol 1990;20:213–35.
51. Gary AT, Kerl ME, Wiedmeyer CE, et al. Bone marrow hypoplasia associated with fenbendazole administration in a dog. J Am Anim Hosp Assoc 2004;40: 224–9.
52. Malik R, Medeiros C, Wigney DI, et al. Suspected drug eruption in seven dogs during administration of flucytosine. Aust Vet J 1996;74:285–8.
53. Webb CB, Twedt DC. Acute hepatopathy associated with mitotane administration in a dog. J Am Anim Hosp Assoc 2006;42:298–301.
54. Rottman JB, English RV, Breitschwerdt EB, et al. Bone marrow hypoplasia in a cat treated with griseofulvin. J Am Vet Med Assoc 1991;198:429–31.
55. Shelton GH, Grant CK, Linenberger ML, et al. Severe neutropenia associated with griseofulvin therapy in cats with feline immunodeficiency virus infection. J Vet Intern Med 1990;4:317–9.
56. Brazzell JL, Weiss DJ. A retrospective study of aplastic pancytopenia in the dog: 9 cases (1996-2003). Vet Clin Pathol 2006;35:413–7.

57. Kunkle GA, Meyer DJ. Toxicity of high doses of griseofulvin in cats. J Am Vet Med Assoc 1987;191:322–3.

58. Stokol T, Randolph JF, Nachbar S, et al. Development of bone marrow toxicosis after albendazole administration in a dog and cat. J Am Vet Med Assoc 1997; 210:1753–6.

Adverse Drug Reactions in Veterinary Patients Associated with Drug Transporters

Katrina L. Mealey, DVM, PhD

KEYWORDS

- ATP-binding cassette transporters • ABCB1 • ABCG2 • Solute carrier
- Pharmacogenetics

KEY POINTS

- Because drug transporters play an important role in drug absorption, distribution, and excretion, alterations in drug transporter function can result in adverse drug reactions.
- The ABCB1 polymorphism in dogs and drug interactions involving P-glycoprotein can enhance the toxicity of many drugs.
- The species-wide ABCG2 defect in cats is responsible for fluoroquinolone-induced retinal toxicity.
- Because drug transporters play an important role in drug disposition, a thorough understanding of drug transporters in companion animals is critical in drug discovery and development.

INTRODUCTION

Most veterinarians consider an adverse drug reaction to be something that happens when excessive drug accumulation results in drug toxicity. Another type of adverse drug event, lack of efficacy, occurs when a drug fails to reach effective concentrations at the site of action. Both types of adverse drug events (lack of drug efficacy or drug toxicity) can be deleterious to the patient, so both should be avoided. Optimal drug therapy is achieved when drugs reach effective concentrations at the site of action but do not reach toxic concentrations in susceptible tissues.

Any factor that influences plasma and/or tissue drug concentrations will influence the optimization of drug therapy. Some obstacles to achieving optimal drug therapy have been discussed in previous articles. Alterations in the function of drug-metabolizing enzymes, whether due to genetic polymorphisms or drug-drug

Disclosures: Dr Mealey and Washington State University hold the patent for MDR1 genotyping and receive royalties for MDR1 genotyping services.
Department of Veterinary Clinical Sciences, College of Veterinary Medicine, Washington State University, Pullman, WA 99164-6610, USA
E-mail address: kmealey@vetmed.wsu.edu

interactions, can increase or decrease plasma and tissue drug concentrations. Other factors that may influence plasma and tissue drug concentrations include liver disease, renal disease, patient age, dietary interactions, and interactions with nondrug supplements such as herbals and so-called nutraceuticals (nutritional supplements).

For many drugs used in veterinary practice, plasma and tissue concentrations are also highly dependent on the activity of drug transporters. These transporters are large transmembrane proteins that function as either drug efflux or uptake pumps.[1] The transporters are expressed to some degree on a variety of tissues while being highly expressed on the surface of tissues that are responsible for drug absorption, metabolism, and excretion, such as liver, intestinal lumen, biliary canaliculi, and renal tubular epithelium.[2] In addition, these transporters are expressed on the endothelium of "sanctuary" or protected sites, including brain, retina, testes, and placenta (**Fig. 1**).[3,4]

Two superfamilies of drug transport proteins are considered to be of major importance in determining drug disposition in human patients: the adenosine triphosphate (ATP)-binding cassette (ABC) superfamily and the solute carrier (SLC) superfamily. Research in human patients and/or knockout mice models have demonstrated clinically significant changes in drug disposition resulting from altered function of these drug transporters.[4] Although specific examples of drug transporter defects in veterinary species are scarce, those that have been documented dramatically illustrate the importance of the ABC transporter family in drug disposition. Altered function of drug transporters either intrinsically (ie, genetic polymorphisms) or extrinsically (ie, drug-drug interactions) can result in decreased drug efficacy or increased risk of toxicity in affected patients. Whether one can extrapolate data from human or mouse studies and apply it to other species depends on the specific transporter and drug involved, because there may be species differences in tissue expression and/or substrate specificity of the transporter.

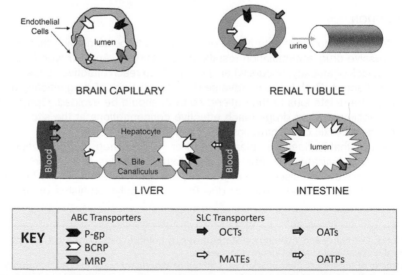

Fig. 1. Major drug transporters of the ABC and SLC superfamilies, their tissue localization, and direction of drug transport. ABC, ATP-binding cassette; BCRP, breast cancer resistance protein; MATEs, multidrug and toxin extrusion transporters; MRP, multidrug resistance–related protein; OATs, organic anion transporters; OATPs, organic anion–transporting polypeptides; OCTs, organic cation transporters; P-gp, P-glycoprotein; SLC, solute carrier.

This article describes how functional changes in drug transporters, whether mediated by genetic variability or drug-drug interactions, affect drug disposition and, ultimately, drug safety and efficacy in veterinary patients. A greater understanding of species, breed, and individual (genetic) differences in drug transporter function, as well as drug-drug interactions involving drug transporters, will result in improved strategies for drug design and will enable veterinarians to incorporate individualized medicine in their practices.

ATP-BINDING CASSETTE SUPERFAMILY

There are more than 40 members of the ABC protein superfamily. These proteins use ATP to transport substrates across biological membranes (often against steep concentration gradients). Substrates for ABC transporters include ions, peptides, hormones, conjugated metabolites, and xenobiotics, including drugs.[1] Only 3 members of the ABC transporter superfamily are known to transport drug molecules as their substrates: P-glycoprotein (P-gp) (encoded by the ABCB1, formerly MDR1, gene); breast cancer resistance protein (BCRP) (encoded by the ABCG2 gene); and multidrug resistance–related protein (MRP) (encoded by the ABCC1 gene).[4] The ABC drug transporters P-gp, BCRP, and MRP are membrane-spanning proteins that function as transmembrane efflux pumps. One or more of these proteins are normally expressed by a variety of mammalian tissues that serve as barriers to drug absorption (apical border of intestinal epithelial cells), and enhance drug elimination from the body (biliary canalicular or renal tubular epithelial cells) or on capillary endothelial cells at so-called sanctuary sites (blood-brain barrier, blood-retina barrier, testes, placenta). Because of their strategic locations and their ability to prevent drug absorption, enhance drug excretion, and prevent drug entry into specialized tissues, it is presumed that ABC drug transporters provide a protective role for the organism by decreasing exposure to potentially toxic xenobiotics. Thus it is not surprising that deficient ABC transporter function can result in significantly enhanced exposure to substrate drugs. Animals with defects in an ABC transporter experience extreme drug sensitivity when exposed to drugs that are substrates for the defective transporter.

ABCB1 (P-Glycoprotein)

P-gp was the first ABC transporter characterized, and is well known for its ability to modulate multidrug resistance in cancer cells in many species.[5] P-gp substrates include many anticancer drugs (anthracyclines, vinca alkaloids, epipodophyllotoxins), macrocyclic lactones (ivermectin, selamectin, milbemycin, and so forth), loperamide, acepromazine, butorphanol, ondansetron, and dozens of other drugs.[4] Several studies have addressed P-gp's role in drug absorption, distribution, and excretion, and how these pharmacokinetic parameters affect safety and efficacy of P-gp substrate drugs in dogs. Much of this information has been generated from studies and clinical observations of dogs affected by a mutation in the ABCB1 (MDR1) gene. The ABCB1 polymorphism in dogs consists of a 4-base-pair deletion mutation. This deletion results in a shift of the reading frame that generates several premature stop codons. Because protein synthesis is terminated before even 10% of the protein product is synthesized, dogs with 2 mutant alleles exhibit a P-gp null phenotype, similarly to *abcb*1 (mdr1) (−/−) knockout mice.[6] Heterozygous dogs with one mutant allele and one wild-type allele (ABCB1 normal/mutant) have an intermediate phenotype. Affected dogs include many herding breeds (**Table 1**). The frequency of the ABCB1-1Δ mutation is very high in some breeds, with affected dogs displaying the

Table 1
Approximate frequencies (%) of MDR1 genotypes in affected dog breeds[a]

Breed	MDR1(Mutant/ Mutant)	MDR1(Mutant/ Normal)	MDR1(Normal/ Normal)
Australian Shepherd	10	35	55
Australian Shepherd (miniature)	5	45	50
Border Collie	2	5	93
Collie	35	45	20
English Shepherd	0	15	85
German Shepherd	2	8	90
Herding breed mix	1	10	89
Longhaired Whippet	15	50	35
McNab	3	28	70
Mixed breed	3	8	89
Old English Sheepdog	0	7	93
Shetland Sheepdog	2	15	83
Silken Windhound	1	33	66

[a] Represent combined results from several different investigations.
Data from Refs.[7–10,39–41]

"multidrug sensitivity" phenotype. Studies have determined that roughly 75% of collies and 50% of Australian Shepherds in the United States,[7] Europe,[8] Japan,[9] and Australia[10] have at least 1 mutant allele. Thus, an understanding of P-gp's role in drug distribution and elimination is critically important when dogs of these breeds are treated with any drug that might be a substrate for P-gp.

Drug distribution, and therefore the risk of drug toxicity, can be dramatically affected by alterations in P-gp function. Because P-gp is a component of the blood-brain barrier, the blood-testes barrier, and the placenta, distribution of P-gp substrate drugs to these tissues is greatly enhanced in ABCB1(mutant/mutant) dogs and moderately enhanced in ABCB1(mutant/normal) dogs. Macrocyclic lactones such as ivermectin can cause neurologic toxicity in any animal at high doses (>2 mg/kg). ABCB1(mutant/mutant) dogs experience adverse neurologic effects after a single dose of ivermectin (>120 µg/kg) and will experience life-threatening neurologic toxicity at the antiparasitic dose of 300 µg/kg because the defective blood-brain barrier allows ivermectin to accumulate in brain tissue of these animals.[6,11] The concentration of ivermectin in brain tissue of abcb1(−/−) knockout mice is 100 times greater than the concentration of ivermectin in brain tissue of wild-type mice.[12] A similar difference in brain accumulation of ivermectin in ABCB1(mutant/mutant) versus ABCB1(normal/normal) dogs would be expected. It is important that the dose of ivermectin used in commercial heartworm preventive products (6 µg/kg per month) will not cause neurologic toxicity even in ABCB1(mutant/mutant) dogs. Dogs with the ABCB1 mutation also have increased susceptibility to neurologic adverse effects of other macrocyclic lactones (milbemycin, selamectin, and moxidectin) as well as the antidiarrheal drug loperamide. Loperamide is an opioid that is generally devoid of central nervous system (CNS) activity because it is excluded from the brain by P-gp. At routinely used therapeutic doses, loperamide causes profound CNS depression in ABCB1(mutant/ mutant) dogs.[13,14] This effect can be reversed by the opioid antagonist naloxone. Less information is available regarding P-gp and the blood-brain barrier in cats. The author has received anecdotal reports of ivermectin toxicity in cats after therapeutic doses (100–300 µg/kg), but whether the underlying cause is a result of altered P-gp expression or function is not currently known.

P-gp also affects drug excretion. Although P-gp is expressed on both renal tubular cells and biliary canalicular cells, evidence is lacking to support an important role for P-gp with respect to renal drug excretion. On the contrary, studies in different species demonstrate the important role P-gp plays in biliary drug excretion. Altered P-gp function has been shown to dramatically alter the disposition of several P-gp substrate drugs. For example, concurrent administration of a P-gp inhibitor decreases the biliary clearance of doxorubicin (P-gp substrate) in rats, resulting in increased plasma concentrations of doxorubicin.[15] Similarly, administration of verapamil (a P-gp inhibitor) to rats decreased biliary excretion of the P-gp substrate irinotecan by half.[16] Studies comparing biliary excretion of the P-gp substrate ^{99m}Tc-sestamibi in ABCB1(normal/normal) and ABCB1(mutant/mutant) dogs demonstrate that ABCB1(mutant/mutant) dogs are not able to excrete this compound into bile.[17] ^{99m}Tc-sestamibi is essentially undetectable in gallbladders of ABCB1(mutant/mutant) dogs but is highly concentrated in gallbladders of ABCB1(normal/normal) dogs. Diminished biliary drug excretion may play a role in the apparent increased sensitivity of herding breeds to toxicity caused by chemotherapeutic drugs that are P-gp substrates. For example, ABCB1(mutant/mutant) and ABCB1(normal/mutant) dogs are significantly more likely than ABCB1(normal/normal) dogs to develop hematologic toxicity (neutropenia and thrombocytopenia) after treatment with the P-gp substrate vincristine.[18] However, these dogs tolerate cyclophosphamide (a drug that is not a P-gp substrate) at full doses. In dogs, vincristine is eliminated primarily via biliary excretion of parent drug with some urinary excretion of parent drug and metabolites. Therefore, reduced doses of P-gp substrate chemotherapeutic agents including vincristine, doxorubicin, and vinblastine should be given to ABCB1(mutant/mutant) and ABCB1(normal/mutant) dogs to avoid severe toxicity.

ABCG2 (Breast Cancer Resistance Protein)

BCRP is expressed on enterocytes, the canalicular membrane of hepatocytes, proximal renal tubule cells, erythrocytes, and hematopoietic stem cells.[19] It is also expressed on endothelial cells of the brain and retina, where it functions as an important component of the blood-brain barrier and the blood-retina barrier. At these locations BCRP functions in a protective capacity, excreting substrate drugs into the intestinal lumen, bile, and urine, or restricting access of substrate drugs to sensitive brain and retinal tissues. In addition, BCRP is expressed in mammary tissue where it transports substrates into milk.[20] Several polymorphisms in ABCG2 have been described in humans. The most well-characterized polymorphism, ABCG2 421C>A, results in a glutamine (polar) to lysine (nonpolar) amino acid change within an important functional domain, the ATP-binding domain.[21] The ATP-binding domain is critical to protein function because ATP binding supplies the energy to pump substrates against a concentration gradient. ABCG2 expression in affected individuals is decreased and ABCG2 transport capacity is reduced when compared with individuals with the wild-type allele. Compared with patients with wild-type ABCG2, oral bioavailability of topotecan is 1.34-fold greater in patients with the ABCG2 421C>A variant.[22] Human patients with the ABCG2 421C>A variant also experience altered pharmacokinetics and/or increased drug-induced toxicity when administered substrate drugs such as gefitinib, irinotecan, sulfasalazine, and other drugs in comparison with individuals with the wild-type allele.[22] Thus, functional changes in ABCG2 are also likely to have therapeutic implications for veterinary patients.

Whereas canine ABCG2 has not been well characterized, characterization of feline ABCG2 has been described.[23] Feline ABCG2 was sequenced and the consensus amino acid sequence compared with that of 10 other mammalian species, including humans. Four feline-specific amino acid changes in conserved regions of ABCG2 were identified. One of the amino acid changes was similar to the human variant ABCG2 421C>A, in that it occurs within the ATP-binding domain and consists of a glutamate (polar) to methionine (nonpolar) shift. Therefore one would predict a similar defect in ABCG2 function. The effect of these feline-specific amino acid changes on ABCG2 function was assessed using transfection experiments. cDNA constructs for feline and wild-type human ABCG2 were inserted in a pcDNA3 expression vector and expressed in HEK 293 cells. ABCG2 transport function was assessed using 2 standard ABCG2 substrates (mitoxantrone and BODIPY-prazosin). As predicted, feline ABCG2 transport of either substrate was defective when compared with wild-type human ABCG2.[23] These results have several important clinical consequences, particularly when one considers that these amino acid changes appear to affect all cats and do not represent an ABCG2 variant (as is the case in humans). Based on this information, in comparison with other species cats would be expected to exhibit enhanced susceptibility to toxicity of ABCG2 substrate drugs.

For more than 20 years, fluoroquinolone antimicrobials have been used in veterinary patients. Domestic cats experience an unusual, and apparently species-specific, adverse drug reaction associated with fluoroquinolones: acute retinal degeneration and blindness.[24] Fluoroquinolone-induced retinal toxicity was first documented with enrofloxacin, which is structurally similar to the human-approved fluoroquinolone ciprofloxacin. Enrofloxacin received approval from the Food and Drug Administration (FDA) in 1990 for use in cats at an oral dose of 2.5 mg/kg/d. In 1997, a flexible dosing label for enrofloxacin was approved, which consisted of a dose range of 5 to 20 mg/kg, per os, either once daily or as a divided daily dose. Shortly after this flexible dosing label was introduced, veterinarians began diagnosing blindness in cats receiving enrofloxacin, particularly after once-daily administration of doses at the high end of the flexible dose range. In a prospective study, enrofloxacin was administered orally at a dose of 50 mg/kg to 12 cats while 12 cats received saline control. All enrofloxacin-treated cats developed retinal degeneration as early as 3 days after enrofloxacin administration, whereas none of the control cats developed retinal lesions.[25] Histopathologic changes included severe vacuolization progressing to necrosis in the photoreceptor layer, outer nuclear layer, and outer plexiform layer of the retina. Thus, high doses of enrofloxacin are acutely toxic to the retina of cats. Orbifloxacin, another fluoroquinolone approved for use in cats and dogs, also causes retinal damage in cats (www.fda.gov freedom of information summary NADA 141-081).

In human patients, cutaneous photosensitivity is known as one of the more common adverse reactions to fluoroquinolones.[26] When exposed to light, fluoroquinolones generate reactive oxygen species (ROS) that attack cellular lipid membranes, causing tissue damage.[27] With the exception of skin, the organ most susceptible to phototoxicity is the eye, including the retina. Retinal degeneration and blindness can result from extensive phototoxic damage to the retina. Under normal conditions, the retina is protected from photoreactive compounds by the blood-retina barrier.[28,29] The blood-retina barrier consists of both capillary endothelial cell tight junctions and retinal pigment epithelial cell tight junctions, as well as important transporters including ABCG2 that function to prevent distribution of drugs to the retina. ABCG2 is strategically positioned on the luminal membrane of retinal capillary endothelial cells, where it actively transports substrates from the endothelial cell back into the capillary lumen.[28]

Because fluoroquinolones are substrates for ABCG2, the distribution of these drugs to retinal tissues is normally restricted by ABCG2.

Dysfunction of ABCG2 in cats results in a dysfunctional blood-retina barrier. Cats experience accumulation of photoreactive fluoroquinolones in their retina in comparison with other species. Exposure of the retina to light then generates ROS, which create the characteristic retinal degeneration and blindness documented in cats receiving high doses of fluoroquinolones. Defective ABCG2 function in cats may also contribute to their sensitivity to acetaminophen. In dogs and humans, acetaminophen is metabolized primarily by glucuronidation and sulfation to nontoxic metabolites. Cytochrome P450 enzymes, which generate a toxic metabolite (NAPQI), are not involved. Relative to other species, cats have low hepatic levels of uridine diphosphate glucuronyltransferase and are unable to use glucuronidation pathways. Thus, acetaminophen metabolism is shifted to the sulfation pathway. In most species ABCG2 mediates the biliary excretion of acetaminophen sulfate. However, in *abcg*2 knockout mice, biliary excretion of acetaminophen sulfate was negligible.[30] Because feline ABCG2 is also dysfunctional, a similar phenomenon would be expected to occur in cats. This process would result in shunting of acetaminophen metabolism away from sulfation in favor of cytochrome P450–mediated pathways where the toxic metabolite NAPQI is generated. Thus, defective ABCG2 function in cats may help explain enhanced susceptibility of cats to acetaminophen toxicity.

A long list of substrates and inhibitors of ABCG2 already exists, and the list continues to expand. With regard to cancer therapy, important substrates of ABCG2 include mitoxantrone, methotrexate, etoposide, and, of particular interest, many tyrosine kinase inhibitors.[22] Two tyrosine kinase inhibitors (toceranib and masitinib) have recently received FDA approval for the treatment of canine mast cell tumors. Of note, tyrosine kinase inhibitors are reported to be both substrates for and inhibitors of ABCG2. Whether defective ABCG2 function in cats will affect efficacy and/or toxicity of tyrosine kinase inhibitors has yet to be determined.

Inhibitors of ABC Transporters Can Mimic Pharmacogenetically Mediated Adverse Reactions

Because P-gp and ABCG2 contribute to multidrug resistance in patients with cancer, numerous drugs have been developed to inhibit these transporters in an effort to improve outcomes in patients treated with chemotherapy. Clinical trials involving inhibitors of ABC transporters have resulted in unexpected and undesired pharmacokinetic interactions between the inhibiting agents and the chemotherapeutic drugs used for treating patients with cancer. For example, inhibiting agents often block renal and/or biliary excretion of anticancer drugs by the ABC transporter, enhancing their accumulation in plasma and thereby increasing the risk of toxicity (ie, myelosuppression, gastrointestinal adverse effects).[31] Inhibiting ABC transporters not only blocks excretion of drugs but also alters their distribution. Inhibiting P-gp has been shown to enhance brain penetration of substrate drugs (mimicking what is seen in MDR1 mutant/mutant dogs).[32] For example, ketoconazole increases brain penetration of ivermectin in MDR1(normal/normal) dogs, causing neurologic toxicity (author's personal observation). Ketoconazole inhibits biliary excretion of ⁹⁹ᵐTc-sestamibi in MDR1(normal/normal) dogs.[17] For P-gp substrate drugs with a narrow therapeutic index (ie, vincristine, doxorubicin), concurrent administration of a drug that inhibits P-gp function should be avoided. Drugs known to inhibit P-gp function in dogs include ketoconazole, cyclosporine, and spinosad.[33]

While less is known about the clinical consequences of ABCG2 inhibition, caution should be exercised. For example, pharmacologic inhibition of ABCG2 would be expected to enhance retinal accumulation of substrate drugs such as fluoroquinolones. Thus, concurrent administration of a fluoroquinolone and an ABCG2 inhibitor (such as a tyrosine kinase inhibitor) may cause retinal degeneration and blindness in any species.

ABCC1 (Multidrug Resistance-Related Protein)

Like many ABC transporters, ABCC1 expression was first identified in cancer cells that were resistant to multiple chemotherapeutic drugs. Subsequently ABCC1 expression was identified in many normal tissues including lung, testis, kidney, placenta, and muscle. ABCC1 substrates include a variety of structurally diverse compounds, including some of the same drugs transported by P-gp (anthracyclines, vinca alkaloids, and some human immunodeficiency virus–1 protease inhibitors).[34] Endogenous substrates for ABCC1 include oxidized glutathione, cysteinyl leukotrienes, and glucuronide and sulfate conjugates. Expression of MRP1 has been reported in both canine and feline tumor cells, but ABCC1 variants in veterinary species have not been reported.

Despite its similarities to other important ABC drug transporters (eg, tissue expression and substrate specificity), altered ABCC1 function in human patients has not been shown to alter drug disposition in a clinically significant manner. This finding may be due to the fact that ABCC1 polymorphisms identified to date do not result in major disruption to ABCC1 transport function. It is also possible that alternative pathways and overlapping substrate specificity with other ABC transporters mitigates the impact of ABCC1 on drug disposition. However, one human ABCC1 variant (ABCC1 Gly67Val) is significantly associated with doxorubicin-induced cardiomyopathy without evidence of altered doxorubicin pharmacokinetics.[35]

SOLUTE CARRIER SUPERFAMILY

The SLC superfamily of transporters uses several different processes (facilitated diffusion, ion coupling, ion exchange) to transport substrates across biological membranes. Some members of the SLC superfamily are uptake transporters (transport substrates into cells) whereas others are efflux transporters (transport substrates out of cells).[1] In humans and rodents, members of the SLC superfamily mediate transport of a variety of structurally diverse compounds, including endogenous and exogenous substances. There is some overlap of substrates among members of the SLC superfamily in humans and rodents. For example, fluvastatin (a cholesterol-lowering drug) is a substrate for at least 3 different members of the human SLC superfamily.[36] Less is known about substrate specificity of canine and feline SLC transporters. In humans, rodents, and, presumably, dogs and cats, SLC transporters are expressed along the body's functional "barrier" tissues including intestine, brain capillary endothelial cells, placenta, liver, and kidney, as well as other tissues. These strategic locations allow SLC transporters to influence drug absorption, distribution, metabolism, and excretion. Members of the SLC superfamily include organic cation transporters (OCTs), multidrug and toxin extrusion transporters (MATEs), organic anion transporters (OATs), and organic anion–transporting polypeptides (OATPs).

Organic Cation Transporters

Among the organic cation transporters in humans, those that appear to play a major role in drug transport include OCT1 (SLC22A1), OCT2 (SLC22A2), and OCT3 (SL22A3).[37] These proteins function as uptake transporters in the tissues where they are expressed. The highest levels of expression of OCT1 and OCT2 are along the basolateral (capillary side) membranes of hepatocytes and renal proximal tubular cells (see **Fig. 1**). OCT3 is expressed in a greater variety of tissues. Substrates for OCTs include endogenous cations such as creatinine and monoamine neurotransmitters, as well as exogenous cations such as metformin, ondansetron, and cimetidine.

Dysfunction of OCTs as a result of genetic variation can dramatically affect the pharmacokinetics and clinical response of substrate drugs in human patients. OCT1 loss-of-function mutations are associated with higher plasma concentrations and increased clinical effects of ondansetron. OCT1 normally transports ondansetron from the capillary lumen into hepatocytes, where it is metabolically inactivated. Lack of OCT1 transport function results in decreased hepatocellular uptake of ondansetron, decreased metabolic inactivation, and higher plasma concentrations of active drug. Similar alterations in drug disposition can be demonstrated in OCT1(−/−) knockout mice. Pharmacokinetics and pharmacodynamics of metformin, an OCT1 substrate, differ significantly in wild-type mice in comparison with OCT1(−/−) knockout mice.

In terms of common veterinary species, there are few data on the impact of OCTs on drug disposition. Because of the potential importance of drug/xenobiotic transport into cow's milk, initial studies have investigated whether OCTs are expressed in an immortalized bovine mammary epithelial cell line.[38] Based on basolateral to apical transport of the OCT substrate tetraethyl ammonium, and the fact that specific OCT inhibitors blocked the transport of tetraethyl ammonium, the investigators concluded that OCTs were expressed by bovine mammary epithelial cells.

Multidrug and Toxin Extrusion Transporters

Although the existence of a renal efflux transport system has been recognized since the late 1990s, MATE transporters were not specifically described until 2005. Tissues with the highest levels of MATE expression are the kidney (luminal membrane of renal proximal tubule cells) and liver (canalicular membrane of hepatocytes) (see **Fig. 1**). Because many of the substrates and inhibitors for MATE transporters overlap with those for OCTs, isolating and identifying the specific actions of MATE transporters is complex and continues to be the subject of ongoing investigations. Although polymorphism in genes encoding MATE transporters have been identified, the consequences of these polymorphisms in clinical patients have not been described. Plasma concentrations of metformin are greater in Mate1(−/−) mice than in wild-type mice,[36] suggesting that alterations in MATE1 transport function, whether genetically mediated or the result of pharmacologic inhibition, would alter the disposition of substrate drugs.

Organic Anion Transporters

Members of the OAT family of transporters pump substrates against a concentration gradient by harnessing the power of a sodium gradient generated by Na^+/K^+-ATPase.[37] The most important OATs with regard to drug transport are OAT1 and OAT3. These 2 transporters have overlapping substrate specificity, but OAT1 is expressed on the basolateral membrane of proximal renal tubular cells, whereas OAT3 is expressed not only on the basolateral membrane of proximal renal tubular cells but also in the choroid plexus. In the kidney OAT1 and OAT3 are uptake transporters, that is, they transport substrates from blood into renal tubular epithelial cells, thus enhancing renal drug clearance (see **Fig. 1**). OAT substrates include steroid hormones, biogenic amines, and angiotensin-converting enzyme inhibitors. OAT inhibitors include many commonly used drugs such as nonsteroidal anti-inflammatories (NSAIDs) and antimicrobials (many penicillins and fluoroquinolones). Of importance, loop diuretics (eg, furosemide) and thiazide diuretics rely on OATs to reach their site of action on the luminal membrane of renal proximal tubular cells.

There are several drug interactions that occur via inhibition of OAT-mediated renal tubular secretion of substrates. The classic example, involving probenecid and β-lactam antibiotics, occurs when probenecid inhibits OAT-mediated secretion of β-lactam drugs, resulting in decreased clearance (and enhanced area under the curve) of β-lactams. Another example is the potentially life-threatening interaction involving NSAIDs and methotrexate. NSAIDs inhibit OAT-mediated renal excretion of methotrexate, which has resulted in severe myelosuppression in human patients following prolonged exposure to methotrexate.[3] The contribution of protein-binding interactions with these 2 highly protein-bound drugs might also contribute to the potentially life-threatening drug interaction.

The author is not aware of genetic variants in OATs in veterinary species that have been associated with changes in drug disposition. However, functional OATs have been demonstrated in a cultured bovine mammary epithelial cell line, indicating that this transport family may be responsible for secreting xenobiotics into cow's milk.[38]

Organic Anion–Transporting Polypeptides

OATPs transport a variety of endogenous compounds including bile acids, thyroid hormones, and glucuronidated and sulfated hormones. Exogenous substrates of OATPs include rifampicin, methotrexate, metformin, and statins (drugs that are not routinely used in veterinary patients).[36] Clinically relevant polymorphisms of OATP1B1 have been described in human patients. OAT1B1 expression in humans occurs exclusively on the basolateral membrane of hepatocytes, where it transports substrates into hepatocytes (see **Fig. 1**). A loss-of-function polymorphism in OAT1B1 results in decreased uptake of substrates by hepatocytes. For drugs such as the statins, whose site of action is within hepatocytes, individuals with loss-of-function mutations demonstrate a poor response to the lipid-lowering effects of this class of drugs in comparison with patients with wild-type OAT1B1.[36] The author is not aware of any genetic variants of OATPs in veterinary species.

REFERENCES

1. DeGorter MK, Xia CQ, Yang JJ, et al. Drug transporters in drug efficacy and toxicity. Annu Rev Pharmacol Toxicol 2012;52:249–73.
2. Dean M, Annilo T. Evolution of the ATP-binding cassette (ABC) transporter superfamily in vertebrates. Annu Rev Genomics Hum Genet 2005;6:123–42.
3. Cutler MJ, Choo EF. Overview of SLC22A and SLCO families of drug uptake transporters in the context of cancer treatments. Curr Drug Metab 2011;12(8): 793–807.
4. Kerb R. Implications of genetic polymorphisms in drug transporters for pharmacotherapy. Cancer Lett 2006;234(1):4–33.
5. Mealey KL. Therapeutic implications of the MDR-1 gene. J Vet Pharmacol Ther 2004;27(5):257–64.
6. Mealey KL, Bentjen SA, Gay JM, et al. Ivermectin sensitivity in collies is associated with a deletion mutation of the mdr1 gene. Pharmacogenetics 2001;11(8): 727–33.
7. Mealey KL, Meurs KM. Breed distribution of the ABCB1-1Delta (multidrug sensitivity) polymorphism among dogs undergoing ABCB1 genotyping. J Am Vet Med Assoc 2008;233(6):921–4.

8. Gramer I, Leidolf R, Doring B, et al. Breed distribution of the nt230(del4) MDR1 mutation in dogs. Vet J 2011;189(1):67–71.
9. Kawabata A, Momoi Y, Inoue-Murayama M, et al. Canine mdr1 gene mutation in Japan. J Vet Med Sci 2005;67(11):1103–7.
10. Mealey KL, Munyard KA, Bentjen SA. Frequency of the mutant MDR1 allele associated with multidrug sensitivity in a sample of herding breed dogs living in Australia. Vet Parasitol 2005;131(3–4):193–6.
11. Nelson OL, Carsten E, Bentjen SA, et al. Ivermectin toxicity in an Australian Shepherd dog with the MDR1 mutation associated with ivermectin sensitivity in Collies. J Vet Intern Med 2003;17(3):354–6.
12. Schinkel AH, Jonker JW. Mammalian drug efflux transporters of the ATP binding cassette (ABC) family: an overview. Adv Drug Deliv Rev 2003;55(1): 3–29.
13. Sartor LL, Bentjen SA, Trepanier L, et al. Loperamide toxicity in a collie with the MDR1 mutation associated with ivermectin sensitivity. J Vet Intern Med 2004; 18(1):117–8.
14. Mealey KL, Greene S, Bagley R, et al. P-glycoprotein contributes to the blood-brain, but not blood-cerebrospinal fluid, barrier in a spontaneous canine p-glycoprotein knockout model. Drug Metab Dispos 2008;36(6):1073–9.
15. Kiso S, Cai SH, Kitaichi K, et al. Inhibitory effect of erythromycin on P-glycoprotein-mediated biliary excretion of doxorubicin in rats. Anticancer Res 2000; 20(5A):2827–34.
16. Bansal T, Mishra G, Jaggi M, et al. Effect of P-glycoprotein inhibitor, verapamil, on oral bioavailability and pharmacokinetics of irinotecan in rats. Eur J Pharm Sci 2009;36(4–5):580–90.
17. Coelho JC, Tucker R, Mattoon J, et al. Biliary excretion of technetium-99m-sestamibi in wild-type dogs and in dogs with intrinsic (ABCB1-1Delta mutation) and extrinsic (ketoconazole treated) P-glycoprotein deficiency. J Vet Pharmacol Ther 2009;32(5):417–21.
18. Mealey KL, Fidel J, Gay JM, et al. ABCB1-1Delta polymorphism can predict hematologic toxicity in dogs treated with vincristine. J Vet Intern Med 2008; 22(4):996–1000.
19. Robey RW, To KK, Polgar O, et al. ABCG2: a perspective. Adv Drug Deliv Rev 2009;61(1):3–13.
20. Merino G, Jonker JW, Wagenaar E, et al. The breast cancer resistance protein (BCRP/ABCG2) affects pharmacokinetics, hepatobiliary excretion, and milk secretion of the antibiotic nitrofurantoin. Mol Pharmacol 2005;67(5):1758–64.
21. Cusatis G, Gregorc V, Li J, et al. Pharmacogenetics of ABCG2 and adverse reactions to gefitinib. J Natl Cancer Inst 2006;98(23):1739–42.
22. Cusatis G, Sparreboom A. Pharmacogenomic importance of ABCG2. Pharmacogenomics 2008;9(8):1005–9.
23. Ramirez CJ, Minch JD, Gay JM, et al. Molecular genetic basis for fluoroquinolone-induced retinal degeneration in cats. Pharmacogenet Genomics 2011;21(2):66–75.
24. Gelatt KN, van der Woerdt A, Ketring KL, et al. Enrofloxacin-associated retinal degeneration in cats. Vet Ophthalmol 2001;4(2):99–106.
25. Ford MM, Dubielzig RR, Giuliano EA, et al. Ocular and systemic manifestations after oral administration of a high dose of enrofloxacin in cats. Am J Vet Res 2007;68(2):190–202.
26. Mehlhorn AJ, Brown DA. Safety concerns with fluoroquinolones. Ann Pharmacother 2007;41(11):1859–66.

27. Agrawal N, Ray RS, Farooq M, et al. Photosensitizing potential of ciprofloxacin at ambient level of UV radiation. Photochem Photobiol 2007;83(5):1226–36.
28. Asashima T, Hori S, Ohtsuki S, et al. ATP-binding cassette transporter G2 mediates the efflux of phototoxins on the luminal membrane of retinal capillary endothelial cells. Pharm Res 2006;23(6):1235–42.
29. Hornof M, Toropainen E, Urtti A. Cell culture models of the ocular barriers. Eur J Pharm Biopharm 2005;60(2):207–25.
30. Zamek-Gliszczynski MJ, Nezasa K, Tian X, et al. The important role of Bcrp (Abcg2) in the biliary excretion of sulfate and glucuronide metabolites of acetaminophen, 4-methylumbelliferone, and harmol in mice. Mol Pharmacol 2006; 70(6):2127–33.
31. Nobili S, Landini I, Giglioni B, et al. Pharmacological strategies for overcoming multidrug resistance. Curr Drug Targets 2006;7(7):861–79.
32. Choo EF, Leake B, Wandel C, et al. Pharmacological inhibition of P-glycoprotein transport enhances the distribution of HIV-1 protease inhibitors into brain and testes. Drug Metab Dispos 2000;28(6):655–60.
33. Dunn ST, Hedges L, Sampson KE, et al. Pharmacokinetic interaction of the antiparasitic agents ivermectin and spinosad in dogs. Drug Metab Dispos 2011; 39(5):789–95.
34. Leslie EM, Deeley RG, Cole SP. Multidrug resistance proteins: role of P-glycoprotein, MRP1, MRP2, and BCRP (ABCG2) in tissue defense. Toxicol Appl Pharmacol 2005;204(3):216–37.
35. Wojnowski L, Kulle B, Schirmer M, et al. NAD(P)H oxidase and multidrug resistance protein genetic polymorphisms are associated with doxorubicin-induced cardiotoxicity. Circulation 2005;112(24):3754–62.
36. Roth M, Obaidat A, Hagenbuch B. OATPs, OATs and OCTs: the organic anion and cation transporters of the SLCO and SLC22A gene superfamilies. Br J Pharmacol 2012;165(5):1260–87.
37. Fahrmayr C, Fromm MF, Konig J. Hepatic OATP and OCT uptake transporters: their role for drug-drug interactions and pharmacogenetic aspects. Drug Metab Rev 2010;42(3):380–401.
38. Al-Bataineh MM, van der Merwe D, Schultz BD, et al. Cultured mammary epithelial monolayers (BME-UV) express functional organic anion and cation transporters. J Vet Pharmacol Ther 2009;32(5):422–8.
39. Mealey KL, Bentjen SA, Waiting DK. Frequency of the mutant MDR1 allele associated with ivermectin sensitivity in a sample population of collies from the northwestern United States. Am J Vet Res 2002;63(4):479–81.
40. Tappin SW, Goodfellow MR, Peters IR, et al. Frequency of the mutant MDR1 allele in dogs in the UK. Vet Rec 2012;171(3):72.
41. Neff MW, Robertson KR, Wong AK, et al. Breed distribution and history of canine mdr1-1Delta, a pharmacogenetic mutation that marks the emergence of breeds from the collie lineage. Proc Natl Acad Sci U S A 2004;101(32):11725–30.

Antimicrobials, Susceptibility Testing, and Minimum Inhibitory Concentrations (MIC) in Veterinary Infection Treatment

Mark G. Papich, DVM, MS

KEYWORDS

- Antimicrobials • Minimum inhibitory concentration • Susceptibility testing
- Veterinary infection treatment

KEY POINTS

- If a laboratory does not adhere to a public standard, such as Clinical and Laboratory Standards Institute (CLSI), breakpoints may vary and interpretation may be inconsistent.
- The first question for the clinician is whether or not a culture and susceptibility test is needed for treatment.
- Bacterial culture and susceptibility tests are needed if the clinician suspects that the infection may be caused by organisms resistant to the empirically selected "first-tier" drugs.
- It is becoming more common for laboratories to directly measure the minimum inhibitory concentration (MIC) of an organism with an antimicrobial dilution test, rather than disk diffusion tests.
- Resistance and susceptibility are determined by comparing the organism's MIC to the drug's breakpoint as established by the CLSI.
- The next edition of CLSI M31 for veterinary drugs will be divided into one table for veterinary interpretive criteria and a separate table for drugs that still rely on human standards for interpretation.
- The changes and updates in interpretive criteria used to establish breakpoints illustrate the need for laboratories to use only the most updated document available for interpretation and standards.
- Susceptibility tests, even when appropriate standards are used, are not perfect.
- When evaluating a patient that has failed to respond to therapy, one must consider the many factors that contribute to antibiotic failure.

Disclosures: The author is the current Chairholder of the CLSI Veterinary Antimicrobial Susceptibility Testing (VAST) subcommittee.
North Carolina State University, College of Veterinary Medicine, 1060 William Moore Drive, Raleigh, NC 27607, USA
E-mail address: mark_papich@ncsu.edu

INTRODUCTION

Many veterinarians submit culture specimens to a laboratory without great thought about the test procedure or the interpretation. The most important information for the clinician is simply which drugs have an "S" and which ones have an "R." These results then guide their treatment. What really goes into this interpretation?

The standards for interpretation are available from the Clinical and Laboratory Standards Institute (CLSI) (http://www.clsi.org/).[1] Not all laboratories in the United States use CLSI standards. It is a voluntary program. However, if a laboratory does not adhere to a public standard, such as CLSI, breakpoints may vary and interpretation may be inconsistent from laboratory to laboratory, or among different regions of the country.

The collection of the specimen and appropriate handling and transportation is best discussed with microbiologists and diagnostic laboratory staff. Some guidelines were developed by the International Society for Companion Animal Infectious Diseases (ISCAID) and published online,[2] as well as on their Internet site (http://www.iscaid.org/).

TO CULTURE OR NOT TO CULTURE?

The first question for the clinician is whether or not a culture and susceptibility test is needed for treatment. The answer often is "no." The empiric choice for initial treatment can be highly reliable and guidelines are available in a variety of sources.[3,4] Empiric selection should be based on the assumption that the infection is not complicated and the infection is caused by wild-type bacteria. It is critically important at this state to define what is meant by wild-type and non–wild-type bacteria. Wild-type strains of bacteria are those that have an absence of acquired and mutational resistance mechanisms, whereas non–wild-type strains of bacteria are those that have the presence of an acquired or mutational resistance mechanism to the drug in question. Wild-type strains may include bacteria that have inherent resistance to antimicrobials. For example, wild-type anaerobic bacteria are inherently resistant to aminoglycosides by virtue of a lack of an oxygen-dependent drug entry to the bacteria. Gram-negative wild-type bacteria of the Enterobacteriaceae family and *Pseudomonas aeruginosa* are inherently resistant to macrolide antibiotics.

Wild-type strains of bacteria may or may not respond clinically to antimicrobial treatment. Likewise, non–wild-type strains may or may not respond clinically to antimicrobial treatment. The prediction of whether the bacteria will, or will not, respond to treatment is commonly referred to as the "90/60 rule."[5] The 90/60 rule was derived from the observation that, in general, bacteria treated with antimicrobials to which the strain is sensitive will have a favorable therapeutic response in approximately 90% of the patients. On the other hand, when the bacteria are resistant to the antimicrobial administered, despite the susceptibility result, approximately 60% of patients will respond to therapy. In veterinary medicine, we have no data to confirm or challenge the 90/60 rule. The investigators[5] emphasize that these observations apply to immunocompetent patients with infections caused by a single bacteria, when the drug is expected to penetrate to the site of infection adequately. Most clinicians would agree that these cases do not comprise all of their patients. Many patients have polymicrobial infections treated with more than one antibiotic, have pathologic changes that may affect drug distribution (eg, protein-binding changes), have received oral antibiotics that are insufficiently absorbed, are immune-compromised patients, or have infections at sites that are either poorly penetrated or diluted, or for which antibiotics are concentrated (for example, from topical treatment or by tubular concentration before clearance by the kidneys).

WHEN IS IT TIME TO CULTURE?

Bacterial culture and susceptibility tests are needed if the clinician suspects that the infection may be caused by organisms resistant to the empirically selected "first-tier" drugs. Without a susceptibility test, the activity against these strains of bacteria is highly unpredictable. Bacteria most likely to be resistant are *Pseudomonas aeruginosa, Escherichia coli, Klebsiella pneumoniae, Enterobacter* species, *Enterococcus* species, and *Staphylococcus pseudintermedius*. A more in-depth discussion of these organisms and their treatment is included in the article "Treatment of Resistant Infections" by M.G. Papich, elsewhere in this issue.

If the initial empiric treatment is unsuccessful, or if resistant strains of bacteria are suspected, a susceptibility test is advised. This test is important to (1) confirm the presence of a bacterial pathogen, (2) identify the species of bacteria so that virulence mechanisms are known, (3) guide treatment, and (4) monitor outcome (success or failure of treatment). Culture and susceptibility tests are advised if the patient has already been exposed to previous antibiotic therapy. Bacteria such as *E coli* are typically more resistant than other species of bacteria. There was a high incidence of resistance in *E coli* isolates collected from different regions of the United States.[6] The multidrug-resistant (MDR) isolates comprised 56% of the resistant isolates and more than half of these were resistant to amoxicillin, amoxicillin-clavulanate, and enrofloxacin. Previous antibiotic treatment is a known risk factor for methicillin-resistant *Staphylococcus*, as well as other resistant bacteria.[7–14] Fluoroquinolone activity may be especially unpredictable if the patient has previously been treated with this class of agents. Previous exposure to fluoroquinolones may select for resistant strains of *E coli* in dogs that can persist long after drug treatment has been discontinued.[15]

TYPES OF SUSCEPTIBILITY TESTS
Agar Disk Diffusion Test

Bacterial susceptibility to drugs has traditionally been tested with the agar-disk-diffusion test (ADD), also known as the Kirby-Bauer test. With this test, paper disks impregnated with the drug are placed on an agar plate and the drug diffuses into the agar. Activity of the drug against the bacteria correlates with the diameter of the zone of bacterial inhibition around the disk, measured in millimeters. In this test, a large zone of inhibition corresponds to a high degree of susceptibility. The larger the zone, the more susceptible the bacteria is to the drug in the disk. The size of the zone of inhibition has an inverse correlation to the minimum inhibitory concentration (MIC), but the size of the zone should not be used to derive an MIC value.

The inoculation variables must be well controlled and the test must be performed according to strict procedural guidelines.[1] The precise incubation time (usually 18–24 hours), selection and preparation of the agar, and interfering compounds should be known. The ADD test results are qualitative (that is, it determines only resistant vs sensitive) rather than providing quantitative information. If this test is performed using standardized procedures, it is valuable, even though it may sometimes overestimate the degree of susceptibility.

Microdilution Test for Determination of MIC

It is becoming more common for laboratories to directly measure the MIC of an organism with an antimicrobial dilution test. The test is usually performed by inoculating the wells of a plate with the bacterial culture and dilutions of antibiotics are arranged across the rows. The test is usually performed in modern laboratories using high-throughput plates, but individual tubes or plates can be used for dilution tests also.

Antibiotic drug concentrations are arranged in serial dilutions, with each concentration doubled from lowest to highest in a range. The MIC is not a measure of efficacy, but instead it is simply an in vitro measurement of drug activity and bacterial susceptibility. The lower the MIC value, the more susceptible the isolate is to that drug. The MICs are determined using serial twofold dilutions of drug to which is added a standardized inoculum that is incubated for a prescribed time. Concentrations are always listed in μg/mL. For example, if one were to start at a concentration of 256 μg/mL, the MIC dilution series would be as follows: 128, 64, 32, 16, 8, 4, 2, 1, 0.5, 0.25, 0.12, 0.06 μg/mL, and so forth. If, for example, bacterial growth occurs at a dilution of 0.12 μg/mL for a specific drug, but not at 0.25 μg/mL and above, the MIC is determined to be 0.25 μg/mL. Realistically, the true MIC lies somewhere between these values, but the MIC is recorded as the next highest value. Like the ADD test, the dilution test should be performed according to strict procedural standards, including quality control, such as those in CLSI documents M31.[1]

In some laboratories, other methods to measure the MIC are being used, such as the E-test (epsilometer test) by bioMérieux SA (bioMérieux, F-69280 Marcy l'Etoile, France, http://www.biomerieux-diagnostics.com). The E-test is a quantitative technique that measures the MIC by direct measurement of bacterial growth along a concentration gradient of the antibiotic contained in a test strip.

WHY REPORT ONLY THE MIC?

The MIC is the lowest concentration that inhibits visible bacterial growth. Frequently this is expressed as MIC_{50} or MIC_{90}, which is the MIC that inhibits 50% or 90% of the bacteria, respectively. It is sometimes cited in error that the MIC_{50} and MIC_{90} are the average concentrations for 50% and 90% efficacy. These values should not be confused with clinical efficacy (more on that later).

The MBC is the Minimum Bactericidal Concentration, which is the lowest concentration that kills 99.9% of the bacteria. Standards are available to measure the MBC, but the test is more complicated and difficult to perform than the MIC determination. Therefore, the MBC is rarely measured or reported in clinical laboratories.

The MPC is the Mutant Prevention Concentration. This is lowest antibiotic concentration that prevents growth of the least-susceptible first-step resistant mutant among a large bacterial population (eg, 10^7 or 10^{10} colony-forming units).[16] It also may be defined as the MIC of the most resistant first-step cell present in a bacterial population. The mutant selection window (MSW) is the concentration between the MIC of susceptible organisms, and the MPC. The MPC test is not standardized and is more difficult to perform in a clinical laboratory. Large inoculums are required. The interpretation of the MPC value for clinical dose determinations is difficult and has not been established for veterinary antimicrobials.

INTERPRETATION OF SUSCEPTIBILITY TESTS

Resistance and susceptibility are determined by comparing the organism's MIC to the drug's breakpoint as established by the CLSI, formerly known as the National Committee for Clinical Laboratory Standards (NCCLS).[1] An example of approved breakpoints is provided in **Table 1**. After a laboratory determines an MIC, it may use the CLSI "SIR" classification for breakpoints (S, susceptible; I, intermediate; or R, resistant). In practice, if the MIC for the bacterial isolate falls in the *susceptible category*, there is a greater likelihood of successful treatment (cure) than if the isolate were classified as resistant. It does not ensure success; drug failure is still possible owing to other drug or patient factors (for example, immune status, immaturity, or severe illness

Table 1
Susceptibility breakpoints for antimicrobials used in animals (CLSI M31-A3, 2008)

Antimicrobial	Susceptible (μg/mL)[a]	Resistant (μg/mL)[a]
Amikacin	≤16[b]	≥64
Ampicillin	≤0.25	≥0.5
Amoxicillin/Clavulanate	≤0.25/0.12	≥1/0.5
Cefazolin	≤2	≥8
Cefotaxime	≤8[b]	≥64
Cefpodoxime	≤2	≥8
Cephalothin[c]	≤2	≥8
Chloramphenicol	≤8[b]	≥32
Cefoxitin	≤8[b]	≥32
Ciprofloxacin	≤1[b]	≥4
Clindamycin	≤0.5	≥4
Difloxacin	≤0.5	≥4
Enrofloxacin	≤0.5	≥4
Erythromycin	≤0.5[b]	≥8
Gentamicin	≤2 (≤500 for Enterococci)	≥8 (≥500 for Enterococci)
Imipenem	≤1[b]	≥4
Marbofloxacin	≤1	≥4
Orbifloxacin	≤1	≥8
Oxacillin (veterinary)	≤0.25	≥0.5
Penicillin G (equine)	≤0.5	≥2.0
Rifampin	≤1[b]	≥4
Tetracycline[d]	≤4[b]	≥16
Ticarcillin	≤64 (*Pseudomonas*)[b] ≤16 (for others)[b]	≥128 ≥128
Trimethoprim/Sulfa	≤2/38[b]	≥4/76
Vancomycin	≤2 (Staphylococci)[b]	≥16 (Staphylococci)

[a] Values between the susceptible and resistant range are interpreted as "intermediate."
[b] Some of the breakpoints listed are derived from human standards listed in M100.
[c] Cephalothin is used to test for other first-generation cephalosporins (eg, cephalexin).
[d] Tetracycline is used to test for other tetracyclines (doxycycline and minocycline).
Data from Clinical Laboratory Standards Institute. Performance standards for antimicrobial disk and dilution susceptibility tests for bacteria isolated from animals. Approved Standard. 3rd edition. CLSI document M31-A3. Wayne (PA): Clinical and Laboratory Standards Institute; 2008.

that compromises the action of antibacterial drugs), and interactions. If the MIC is in the *resistant category*, bacteriologic failure is more likely because of specific resistance mechanisms or inadequate drug concentrations in the patient. However, a patient with a competent immune system may sometimes eradicate an infection even when the isolate is resistant to the drug in the MIC test.

The *intermediate category* is intended as a buffer zone between susceptible and resistant strains. This category reflects the possibility of error when an isolate has an MIC that borders between susceptible and resistant. If the MIC value is in the intermediate category, therapy with this drug at the usual standard dosage is discouraged because there is a good likelihood that drug concentrations may be inadequate for a cure. However, successful therapy is possible when drug concentrates at certain sites (in urine, or as the result of topical therapy, for example) or at doses higher than the minimum effective dose listed on the label. Prescribing guidelines for some antimicrobials allow for an increase in dose when susceptibility testing identifies an organism in the intermediate range of susceptibility. For example, fluoroquinolone antimicrobials have been approved with a dose range that allows increases in doses when susceptibility testing identifies an organism in the *intermediate* range of susceptibility. In these cases, higher drug concentrations make a cure possible if the clinician is able to safely increase the dose above the minimum labeled dose. (For example, in the case of enrofloxacin in dogs, this would be equivalent to a dose of 10–20 mg/kg/d, rather than the minimum dose of 5 mg/kg/d.)[17]

MIC data should not be used in isolation, but by coupling the MIC from a laboratory report with CLSI breakpoints and other important information, such as the virulence of the bacteria and the pharmacology of the antibiotics being considered, the clinician can make a more informed selection of an antibacterial drug.

Does the Susceptibility Test Provide Tissue-Specific Interpretation?

The susceptibility interpretation is based on plasma/serum concentrations. No tissue-specific interpretation can be provided that accounts for differences in drug distribution among tissues. For example, even though it is anticipated that many antibiotics concentrate in the urine, which may be beneficial for treating a urinary tract infection, the susceptibility interpretation is based on achieving adequate concentrations in the blood. (There are 2 exceptions to this because amoxicillin and amoxicillin-clavulanate interpretations allow for high concentrations in urine.) One should not assume that concentrations in urine, even when they are high due to concentration by the nephrons, are sufficient to eradicate infections of the urinary tract. Infections may involve the deeper layers of the mucosa, the renal tissue, or the prostate tissue. In these instances, it is the tissue concentration, which is correlated to the plasma concentration, that will be predictive of a bacteriologic cure.[18]

A frequent mistake in MIC interpretation is to compare the MIC with published tissue concentrations that are derived from whole-tissue homogenized samples.[19] Tissue concentration data are often published by pharmaceutical companies in their product information. These concentrations may be misleading because they may either underestimate or overestimate (depending on the drug's affinity for intracellular sites) the true drug concentration at the site of infection.

In most instances, the clinician should not be concerned with the question of whether or not there are tissue-specific susceptibility interpretations. For most tissues, antibiotic protein-unbound drug concentrations in the serum or plasma approximate the drug concentration in the extracellular space (interstitial fluid). This is because there is no barrier that impedes drug diffusion from the vascular compartment to extracellular tissue fluid.[20,21] There is really no such thing as "good penetration" and "poor penetration" when referring to most drugs in most tissues. Pores (fenestrations) or microchannels in the endothelium of capillaries are large enough to allow drug molecules to pass through unless the drug is restricted by protein binding in the blood. Tissues lacking pores or channels may inhibit penetration of some drugs (discussed later in this article).

If adequate drug concentrations can be achieved in plasma, it is unlikely that a barrier in the tissue will prevent drug diffusion to the site of infection as long as the tissue has an adequate blood supply. Clinicians should be concerned when treating tissues that have poor or impaired blood supply. Drug diffusion into an abscess or granulation tissue is sometimes a problem, because in these conditions, drug penetration relies on simple diffusion and the site of infection lacks adequate blood supply. In an abscess, there may not be a physical barrier to diffusion (that is, there is no impenetrable membrane) but low drug concentrations are attained in the abscess and drug concentrations may be slow to accumulate.

In some tissues, a lipid membrane (such as tight junctions on capillaries) presents a barrier to drug diffusion. In these instances, a drug must be sufficiently lipid-soluble, or be actively carried across the membrane to reach effective concentrations in tissues. These tissues include the central nervous system, eye, and prostate. A functional membrane pump (p-glycoprotein) also contributes to the barrier. There also is a barrier between plasma and bronchial epithelium (blood-bronchus barrier).[22] This limits drug concentrations of some drugs in the bronchial secretions and epithelial fluid of the airways. Lipophilic drugs may be more likely to diffuse through the blood-bronchus barrier and reach effective drug concentrations in bronchial secretions.

Is Susceptibility Interpretation by CLSI Specific for Veterinary Species?

In past years, the veterinary diagnostic laboratories had to rely heavily on the CLSI interpretation from the human standards. There were not enough veterinary-specific interpretive criteria available to establish breakpoints for veterinary drugs and veterinary species. This is now changing. The next edition of CLSI M31 for veterinary drugs will be divided into 2 tables: one table for veterinary interpretive criteria, and a separate table for drugs that still rely on human standards for interpretation. In the past several years, CLSI has tremendously expanded the list of drugs for which there are veterinary-specific breakpoints. For companion animals, veterinary-specific MIC breakpoints have now been established for the 4 licensed fluoroquinolones: enrofloxacin, difloxacin, marbofloxacin, and orbifloxacin, but not ciprofloxacin. There are also veterinary breakpoints for gentamicin, cefpodoxime proxetil, ampicillin/amoxicillin, amoxicillin-clavulanic acid, first-generation cephalosporins (cephalexin and cefazolin), and clindamycin (dogs only). Important changes were also made for the interpretation of *Staphylococcus* resistance. This is illustrated in more detail later in this article. Until other veterinary-specific breakpoints are established for other antibiotics used in companion animals, we will continue to rely on the human breakpoints for drugs such as amikacin, chloramphenicol, erythromycin, carbapenems (imipenem), penicillins, sulfonamides, potentiated sulfonamides, and tetracyclines. Revised breakpoints for some of these drugs may be available in the next year. But in the meantime, similarities in pharmacokinetics and pathogen susceptibilities between humans and animals allow for an acceptable approximation to extrapolate human breakpoints to animal situations for many drugs until veterinary-specific standards are available.

Veterinary-specific testing issues for Staphylococcus
The previous standards published by the CLSI (CLSI M31-A3, 2008) did not differentiate the interpretive criteria of *Staphylococcus aureus* from that of *Staphylococcus pseudintermedius or Staphylococcus intermedius*; however, this has been corrected in the new edition (M31-A4) to be published in 2013. This edition will indicate that the *S aureus* interpretive criteria uses an MIC breakpoint of greater than or equal to 4.0 µg/mL to define resistance. However, for non–*S aureus* isolates from animals, *Staphylococcus* spp should be considered resistant when the MIC is greater than or equal to 0.5 µg/mL. This interpretation differentiates *S pseudintermedius* from *S aureus*.[23] The current CLSI standard instructs laboratories to report non–*S aureus* isolates from animals that are oxacillin resistant as positive for *mecA*, or that produce PBP 2a, the *mecA* gene product. Laboratories should report *mecA*-positive and/or PBP 2a producing methicillin-resistant *Staphylococcus* as resistant to all other penicillins, carbapenems, cephalosporins (cephems), and β-lactam/β-lactamase inhibitor combinations, regardless of in vitro test results with those agents.

If the previous criteria of greater than or equal to 4.0 μg/mL is used, resistant staph-ylococci from animals may be misidentified. In the next published supplement of the CLSI standards, this recommendation will change to reflect this new evidence. Until then, diagnostic laboratories should adopt the recommendation that if any non-*aureus* coagulase-positive *Staphylococcus* isolated from animals has an MIC value greater than or equal to 0.5 μg/mL (corresponding to a zone diameter of ≤17 mm), it should be considered methicillin resistant, *mec-A* positive, and resistant to all β-lactam anti-biotics. The cefoxitin disk is no longer recommended for testing *S pseudintermedius*, as it was in older editions of CLSI M31.

The need for current standards

These changes and updates in the interpretive criteria used to establish breakpoints illustrate the need for laboratories to use only the most updated document available for interpretation and standards. The previous edition of CLSI-VAST M31[1] will be replaced by a new supplement in 2013. Human breakpoints also are being revised. Because of concerns for misidentifying extended-spectrum β-lactamase–producing Enterobacteriaceae, the cephalosporin breakpoints have been lowered compared with previous criteria.[24,25] Carbapenem breakpoints also have been recently lowered.

HOW ARE BREAKPOINTS DERIVED?

The CLSI subcommittee for Veterinary Antimicrobial Susceptibility Testing (VAST) uses strict criteria to establish and evaluate breakpoints. Sponsors are required to follow guidelines provided by CLSI and must submit data to support a proposed breakpoint. The data include pharmacokinetic data in the target species, MIC distribu-tions for the pathogens targeted, clinical data from the drug used under field condi-tions at the approved dose, and pharmacokinetic-pharmacodynamic (PK-PD) analysis, using Monte Carlo simulations[26] to show that at the approved dose the drug attains PK-PD targets for the labeled pathogen.[27]

ARE THESE STANDARDS, OR GUIDELINES?

The CLSI is a consensus-driven process and after approval by the subcommittee the standards become public documents. The consensus process involves the develop-ment and public open review of documents, revision of documents in response to dis-cussion, and, finally, the acceptance of a document as a consensus standard or guideline. The CLSI M31 document used for culture and susceptibility testing[1] should be regarded as a public standard, not a guideline.

A *standard* is a document developed through the consensus process that clearly identifies specific, essential requirements for materials, methods, or practices for use in an unmodified form. A standard may, in addition, contain discretionary elements, which are clearly identified.

A *guideline* is a document developed through the consensus process describing criteria for a general operating practice, procedure, or material for voluntary use. A guideline may be used as written or modified by the user to fit specific needs.

PITFALLS OF SENSITIVITY TESTING

Susceptibility tests, even when appropriate standards are used, are not perfect. The 90/60 rule discussed earlier reminds us that we are treating animals with uncertain underlying disease and immune status. Individual animals may vary in the drug phar-macokinetics, response to treatment, and immune status. There are many reasons

> **Box 1**
> **Reasons for antimicrobial failure**
>
> - Incorrect diagnosis.
> - Incorrect dose, route, frequency of administration.
> - Depressed patient immunologic status.
> - Poor owner compliance.
> - Antibacterial drug resistance.
> - Presence of pus and a foreign body.[28]
> - Presence of a biofilm.[29,30]
> - Pharmacokinetic drug interactions.
> - Antibiotic antagonism.
> - Pharmacokinetic problems: poor oral absorption, pharmacokinetic antagonism, intestinal metabolism of drug.

why susceptibility tests may not accurately predict an outcome. Among these are the following:

Susceptibility tests assume equal plasma and tissue concentrations. As indicated earlier, a susceptibility test will *over*estimate the antimicrobial activity in tissues difficult to penetrate, such as the central nervous system, prostatic fluid, eye, and respiratory tract. On the other hand, susceptibility tests *under*estimate activity of topical treatments, local infusions, and antibacterials that concentrate in the urine.

Susceptibility tests underestimate activity at concentrations below MIC (sub-MIC). Some drugs exhibit antibacterial effects at concentrations below the MIC, but this cannot be measured under the conditions of the usual susceptibility tests.

Susceptibility tests usually do not test for antibiotic combinations and may miss potentially synergistic combinations (exceptions that are measured include trimethoprim-sulfonamides and amoxicillin-clavulanate).

Susceptibility tests cannot consider the local factors that may affect antimicrobial activity, such as pus, low oxygen tension, or poor blood flow to tissue.

There are not standards available for interpretation of all veterinary-specific drugs. Human standards are used for interpretation for many drugs and may not be equivalent.

Veterinarians are quick to attribute an unsuccessful antimicrobial treatment to a failure of the culture and susceptibility test. There are many reasons why antimicrobial treatment fails. When evaluating a patient that has failed to respond to therapy, one must consider any of the many factors that contribute to antibiotic failure, such as the factors listed in **Box 1**.

REFERENCES

1. Clinical Laboratory Standards Institute (CLSI). Performance standards for antimicrobial disk and dilution susceptibility tests for bacteria isolated from animals. Approved Standard—3rd edition. Wayne (PA): Clinical and Laboratory Standards Institute; 2008. CLSI document M31–A3.
2. Weese JS, Blondeau JM, Boothe D, et al. Antimicrobial use guidelines for treatment of urinary tract disease in dogs and cats: Antimicrobial Guidelines Working

Group of the International Society for Companion Animal Infectious Diseases. Vet Med Int 2011;2011:263768.

3. Papich MG. Handbook of antimicrobial therapy for small animals. St Louis (MO): Elsevier-Saunders; 2011. p. 140.

4. Papich MG. Saunders handbook of veterinary drugs. 3rd edition. St Louis (MO): Elsevier-Saunders; 2011. p. 858.

5. Doern GV, Brecher SM. The clinical predictive value (or lack thereof) of the results of in vitro antimicrobial susceptibility tests. J Clin Microbiol 2011;49(Suppl 9): S11–4.

6. Shaheen BW, Boothe DM, Oyarzabal OA, et al. Antimicrobial resistance profiles and clonal relatedness of canine and feline *Escherichia coli* pathogens expressing multidrug resistance in the United States. J Vet Intern Med 2010;24:323–30.

7. Baker SA, Van-Balen J, Lu B, et al. Antimicrobial drug use in dogs prior to admission to a veterinary teaching hospital. J Am Vet Med Assoc 2012;241:210–7.

8. Gibson JS, Morton JM, Cobbold RN, et al. Multi-drug resistant *E. coli* and *Enterobacter* extraintestinal infection in 37 dogs. J Vet Intern Med 2008;22:844–50.

9. Weese JS, Faires MC, Frank LA, et al. Factors associated with methicillin-resistant versus methicillin-susceptible *Staphylococcus pseudintermedius* infection in dogs. J Am Vet Med Assoc 2012;240(12):1450–5.

10. Petersen AD, Walker RD, Bowman MM, et al. Frequency of isolation and antimicrobial susceptibility patterns of *Staphylococcus intermedius* and *Pseudomonas aeruginosa* isolates from canine skin and ear samples over a 6 year period (1992-1997). J Am Anim Hosp Assoc 2002;38:407–13.

11. Prescott JF, Hanna WJ, Reid-Smith R, et al. Antimicrobial drug use and resistance in dogs. Can Vet J 2002;43:107–16.

12. Martin Barrasa JL, Lupiola Gomez P, Gonzalez Lama Z, et al. Antibacterial susceptibility patterns of *Pseudomonas* strains isolated from chronic canine otitis externa. J Vet Med B Infect Dis Vet Public Health 2000;47:191–6.

13. Oluoch AO, Kim CH, Weisiger RM, et al. Nonenteric *Escherichia coli* isolates from dogs: 674 cases (1990-1998). J Am Vet Med Assoc 2001;218:381–4.

14. Cooke CL, Singer RS, Jang SS, et al. Enrofloxacin resistance in *Escherichia coli* isolated from dogs with urinary tract infections. J Am Vet Med Assoc 2002;220: 190–2.

15. Boothe DM, Debavalya N. Impact of routine antimicrobial therapy on canine fecal *Escherichia coli* antimicrobial resistance: a pilot study. Int J Appl Res Vet Med 2011;9(4):396–406.

16. Epstein BJ, Gums JG, Drlica K. The changing face of antibiotic prescribing: the mutant selection window. Ann Pharmacother 2004;38(10):1675–82.

17. Papich MG, Riviere JE. Chapter 38. Fluoroquinolone antimicrobial drugs. In: Riviere JE, Papich MG, editors. Veterinary pharmacology and therapeutics. 9th edition. Ames (IA): Wiley-Blackwell Publishing; 2009. p. 1524.

18. Frimodt-Møller N. Correlation between pharmacokinetic/pharmacodynamic parameters and efficacy for antibiotics in the treatment of urinary tract infections. Int J Antimicrob Agents 2002;19:546–53.

19. Mouton JW, Theuretzbacher U, Craig WA, et al. Tissue concentrations: do we ever learn? J Antimicrob Chemother 2008;61(2):235–7.

20. Cars C. Pharmacokinetics of antibiotics in tissue and tissue fluids: a review. Scand J Infect Dis Suppl 1991;74:23–33.

21. Nix DE, Goodwin SD, Peloquin CA, et al. Antibiotic tissue penetration and its relevance: impact of tissue penetration on infection response. Antimicrob Agents Chemother 1991;35:1953–9.

22. Kiem S, Schentag JJ. Interpretation of antibiotic concentration ratios measured in epithelial lining fluid. Antimicrob Agents Chemother 2008;52(1):24–36.
23. Bemis DA, Jones RD, Frank LA, et al. Evaluation of susceptibility test breakpoints used to predict mecA-mediated resistance in *Staphylococcus pseudintermedius* isolated from dogs. J Vet Diagn Invest 2009;21(1):53–8.
24. Dudley MN, Ambrose PG, Bhavnani SM, et al, for the Antimicrobial Susceptibility Testing Sub-Committee of the Clinical Laboratory Standards Institute. Background and rationale for revised Clinical Laboratory Standards Institute (CLSI) interpretive criteria (breakpoints) for Enterobacteriaceae and *Pseudomonas aeruginosa*: I. Cephalosporins and Aztreonam. Clin Infect Dis, in press.
25. Kahlmeter G. Breakpoints for intravenously used cephalosporins in Enterobacteriaceae—EUCAST and CLSI breakpoints. Clin Microbiol Infect 2008;14(Suppl 1): 169–74.
26. Ambrose PG. Monte Carlo simulation in the evaluation of susceptibility breakpoints: predicting the future: insights from the Society Of Infectious Diseases Pharmacists. Pharmacotherapy 2006;26(1):129–34.
27. Drusano GL. Pharmacokinetics and pharmacodynamics of antimicrobials. Clin Infect Dis 2007;45(Suppl 1):S89–95.
28. Konig C, Simmen HP, Blaser J. Bacterial concentrations in pus and infected peritoneal fluid—implication of bactericidal activity of antibiotics. J Antimicrob Chemother 1998;42:227–32.
29. Habash M, Reid G. Microbial biofilms: their development and significance for medical device-related infections. J Clin Pharmacol 1999;39:887–98.
30. Smith AW. Biofilms and antibiotic therapy: is there a role for combating resistance by the use of novel drug delivery systems? Adv Drug Deliv Rev 2005;57:1539–50.

Antibiotic Treatment of Resistant Infections in Small Animals

Mark G. Papich, DVM, MS

KEYWORDS

- Antibiotics • Resistance • Infection • Small animals

KEY POINTS

- There are few veterinary clinical studies to support a recommended use and dose for treating drug-resistant infections in small animals and many of these details have been extrapolated from human medicine.
- If the organism is *Pseudomonas aeruginosa*, *Enterobacter* species, *Klebsiella* species, *Escherichia coli*, or *Proteus* species, resistance against many common antibiotics is possible and a susceptibility test is advised using Clinical and Laboratory Standards Institute standards.
- Infections caused by *P aeruginosa* presents a special problem because so few drugs are active against this organism.
- *Staphylococcus* isolated from small animals is most likely to be *Staphylococcus pseudintermedius* rather than *Staphylococcus aureus*.
- The most important resistance mechanism for *Staphylococcus* is methicillin resistance.
- Enterococci are gram-positive cocci that have emerged as important causes of infections, especially those that are nosocomial.
- Isolation of *Enterococcus* species from a site does not always indicate that treatment is needed.
- After a susceptibility report is available, the only antimicrobials to which some gram-negative bacilli are susceptible, including *P aeruginosa*, may be extended-spectrum cephalosporins, carbapenems (penems), selected penicillin derivatives, amikacin, or tobramycin.
- Because susceptibility to non–β-lactam antibiotics is unpredictable, a susceptibility test is needed to identify the most appropriate drug to administer for these infections.
- In response to the emergence of resistant gram-positive bacteria in humans (primarily methicillin-resistant *Staphylococcus* and drug-resistant *Enterococcus* spp) the pharmaceutical industry has responded with new antibiotics for treating these infections in people, but there has not been an equal response in veterinary medicine.

Disclosure: Dr Papich has received consulting fees, research support, and/or gifts from the following companies: Zoetis, Bayer Animal Health, Merck, and Intervet. Dr Papich is the current Chairholder of the Clinical Laboratory Standards Institute (CLSI).
College of Veterinary Medicine, North Carolina State University, 1060 William Moore Drive, Raleigh, NC 27607, USA
E-mail address: mark_papich@ncsu.edu

INTRODUCTION

Treatment guidelines are established in textbooks and consensus documents available for treating routine infections in small animals. Dosage regimens have been established and drug manufacturers have produced several important drugs to treat these common infections encountered in small animals. But these regimens and approved antibiotics for animals are designed for susceptible (wild-type) infections and are often not active against bacteria that carry resistance mechanisms. When the patient has an infection that is refractory to treatment, and/or caused by a resistant organism, other strategies and drugs may be necessary. As with many new treatments, there are few veterinary clinical studies to support a recommended use and dose, and many of these details have been extrapolated from human medicine.

WHAT BACTERIA ARE LIKELY TO BE RESISTANT?
Resistant Gram-negative Bacteria

If the organism is *Pseudomonas aeruginosa*, *Enterobacter* species, *Klebsiella* species, *Escherichia coli*, or *Proteus* species, resistance against many common antibiotics is possible and a susceptibility test is advised using Clinical Laboratory Standards Institute (CLSI) standards.[1] For example, a report showed that among nonenteric *E coli* only 23% were sensitive to a first-generation cephalosporin and less than half were sensitive to ampicillin. In the same study, 13% and 23% were intermediate or resistant to enrofloxacin and orbifloxacin, respectively.[2] In urinary tract infections,[3] half of the *E coli* were resistant to cephalexin, and only 22% were susceptible to enrofloxacin. There was a high incidence of resistance in *E coli* isolates collected from different regions of the United States.[4] The multidrug-resistant (MDR) isolates comprised 56% of the resistant isolates and more than half of these were resistant to amoxicillin, amoxicillin-clavulanate, and enrofloxacin.

P aeruginosa

Infections caused by *P aeruginosa* present a special problem because so few drugs are active against this organism. *P aeruginosa* has an ability to develop resistance via its large genome and multiple mechanisms that produce resistance to the most commonly used antibiotics. Of the β-lactam antibiotics, a few are designated as anti-*Pseudomonas* antibiotics. Although extended-spectrum cephalosporins (second-generation or third-generation cephalosporin) usually are active against enteric gram-negative bacteria, they are not active against *P aeruginosa*. Ceftazidime, an injectable third-generation cephalosporin, is an exception because it has consistently shown activity against *P aeruginosa*.

In one published study, the in vivo activity was examined in 23 strains of *Pseudomonas*: 19 *P aeruginosa*, 3 *Pseudomonas fluorescens* and 1 *Pseudomonas* spp. The most effective antibiotics were tobramycin (100% susceptible), marbofloxacin (91.3%), and ceftazidime (91.3%). Ticarcillin and gentamicin showed good activity (86% and 65.2% respectively). Lower susceptibility was found with enrofloxacin (52.1%).[5] Isolates of *P aeruginosa* from otitis media showed that 97% were susceptible to ceftazidime, and 81% to carbenicillin.[6] Fewer were susceptible to enrofloxacin (51%) and gentamicin (68%). In a study that isolated *P aeruginosa* from the skin and ears of dogs, the pattern of resistance was similar.[7] There were no trends identified, and most isolates were susceptible to ciprofloxacin, piperacillin, ticarcillin, amikacin, and gentamicin (enrofloxacin was not tested). However, isolates from the ears tended to be more resistant than isolates from the skin, with lower susceptibility to topical drugs such as gentamicin.

Staphylococcus Species

Staphylococcus isolated from small animals is most likely to be *Staphylococcus pseudintermedius* rather than *Staphylococcus aureus*. (Previously identified *Staphylococcus intermedius* probably have been misidentified and are now referred to as *S pseudintermedius* by most laboratories.) When infection is caused by a typical wild-type strain, *S pseudintermedius* has a predictable susceptibility to β-lactamase–resistant β-lactam antibiotics such as amoxicillin combined with a β-lactamase inhibitor (Clavamox), a first-generation cephalosporin such as cephalexin or cefadroxil, or the third-generation cephalosporins cefovecin (Convenia) and cefpodoxime (Simplicef). *Staphylococcus* is also susceptible to oxacillin and dicloxacillin (even though these are not used commonly in small animal medicine). Previous reports of studies on *S pseudintermedius* have shown that, despite frequent use in small animals of the drugs mentioned earlier, the distribution of wild-type strains has remained consistent.[8,9] However, methicillin-resistant *Staphylococcus* species, especially *S pseudintermedius*, are being isolated with increased frequency from animals with skin infections.[10–12] These infections are not confined to dermatology. Orthopedic surgeons have also encountered these strains as a cause of postsurgical orthopedic infections.

Resistant mechanisms

The most important resistance mechanism for *Staphylococcus* is methicillin resistance. Methicillin resistance presents a problem for veterinarians because, in addition to resistance to β-lactam antibiotics, most of these bacteria are also multidrug resistant. Staphylococcal methicillin resistance is caused by acquisition of the *mecA* gene, which encodes an altered penicillin-binding protein (PBP-2a). Although oxacillin is used as the surrogate for testing, these are referred to as methicillin-resistant staphylococci.[13–17] Methicillin has replaced oxacillin for testing in laboratories and resistance to oxacillin is equivalent to methicillin resistance. If the pathogen is *S aureus*, the term methicillin-resistant *S aureus* (MRSA) can be applied. However, *S aureus* is an infrequent pathogen in dogs, and is only occasionally found in cats. Bacteria from dogs and cats are most likely *S pseudintermedius* and these strains are referred to as methicillin-resistant *S pseudintermedius* (MRSP).[18,19] Other *Staphylococcus* species also have been identified among veterinary isolates, including coagulase-negative *Staphylococcus*.

If staphylococci are resistant to oxacillin or methicillin, they should be considered resistant to all other β-lactams, including cephalosporins and amoxicillin-clavulanate (eg, Clavamox), regardless of the susceptibility test result. Adding a β-lactamase inhibitor does not overcome methicillin resistance. However, these bacteria often carry coresistance to many other non–β-lactam drugs, including lincosamides (clindamycin, lincomycin), fluroquinolones, macrolides (erythromycin), tetracyclines, and trimethoprim-sulfonamides. In the report by Bemis and colleagues,[17] more than 90% of the methicillin-resistant isolates of *S pseudintermedius* also were resistant to more than 4 other drugs. The cause of the increased frequency of resistance has not been identified with certainty. Use of fluoroquinolones and cephalosporins in people has been linked to emergence of methicillin-resistant *S aureus*.[20–22]

Resistant Enterococcus

Enterococci are gram-positive cocci that have emerged as important causes of infections, especially those that are nosocomial. The most common species identified are *Enterococcus faecalis* and *Enterococcus faecium*. *E faecalis* is more common, but *E faecium* is usually the more resistant. Wild-type strains of enterococci may still be susceptible to penicillin G and ampicillin, or amoxicillin, which is ordinarily the preferred first choice. However, the enterococci have an inherent resistance to cephalosporins and fluoroquinolones. These strains also are usually resistant to trimethoprim-sulfonamide combinations, clindamycin, and macrolides (erythromycin). Susceptibility test results for cephalosporins, β-lactamase–resistant penicillins (eg, oxacillin), trimethoprim-sulfonamide combinations, and clindamycin can give misleading results.[1] Even if isolates are shown to be susceptible to a fluoroquinolone, this class of drugs may not be a good alternative for treatment.

In human medicine, frequent use of fluoroquinolones and cephalosporins (both of which have poor activity against enterococci) has been attributed to emergence of a higher rate of enterococcal infections.[22] Evidence to document this trend is limited in veterinary medicine, but one study from a veterinary teaching hospital indicated an increased rate of enterococcal urinary tract infections.[23]

Isolation of *Enterococcus* species from a site does not always indicate that treatment is needed. If there is no evidence of clinical signs, such as asymptomatic bacteriuria, treatment may be withheld and the patient simply monitored. The low pathogenicity of *Enterococcus* may not justify the risks and expense of antibiotic treatment. When enterococci are present in wound infections, lower urinary tract, peritoneal infections, and body cavity infections (eg, peritonitis), the organism may exist with other bacteria such as gram-negative bacilli or anaerobic bacteria. In these cases, there is evidence that treatment should be aimed at the anaerobe and/or gram-negative bacilli and not directed at the *Enterococcus*. Treatment cures are possible if the other organisms are eliminated without specific therapy for *Enterococcus*.[24]

If treatment is needed, selection of the appropriate agent for *Enterococcus* is frustrating because there are so few drug choices. If possible, the clinician should be guided by a valid culture and susceptibility test performed using the standards listed by the CLSI.[1] If the *Enterococcus* isolated is sensitive to a penicillin, amoxicillin or ampicillin should be administered at the high -end of the dose range. When possible, combine an aminoglycoside with a β-lactam antibiotic for treating serious infections. One of the carbapenems (imipenem-cilastatin) or an extended-spectrum penicillin (eg, piperacillin) can occasionally be considered for treatment of *E faecalis* (but not *E faecium*).

For resistant strains, selecting the appropriate antibiotic is difficult because of the unpredictable nature of these strains. As mentioned later, sometimes the only active drug is chloramphenicol, a glycopeptide (vancomycin), or the oxazolidinone linezolid. Dosage regimens and problems associated with these agents have been discussed in other sources.[25–27]

DRUG CHOICES FOR RESISTANT GRAM-NEGATIVE INFECTIONS

A susceptibility report may show that the only antimicrobials to which some gram-negative bacilli, including *P aeruginosa*, are susceptible are extended-spectrum cephalosporins, carbapenems (penems), selected penicillin derivatives, amikacin, or tobramycin.

Cephalosporins

When injectable cephalosporins are considered for resistant infections in small animals, those most often used are cefotaxime and ceftazidime, although individual veterinary hospitals have used others in this group. Ceftriaxone is a commonly used third-generation cephalosporin in people. It has high protein binding in people (95%), and a long half-life (8 hours) that allows once-daily convenient dosing. However, the protein binding in dogs is lower (25%) and the short half-life (approximately

1 hour) does not confer any advantage compared with other drugs in this group. Ceftiofur is popular for use in large animals, but is not suitable for resistant infections in small animals. Its only approval in small animals is for urinary tract infections in dogs. Effective concentrations are attained only in urine, and high doses can produce adverse effects in dogs.

In general, the third-generation cephalosporins are expensive, and must be injected. These drugs are usually given via the intravenous (IV) route, although subcutaneous (SC), and intramuscular (IM) routes have been used. As with the penicillins, frequent administration is necessary (for example, every 6–8 hours in animals with normal kidney function) because of their time-dependent activity and short half-lives. Dosage regimens have been published in other sources.[25,26] Of the cephalosporins, only the third-generation cephalosporins, ceftazidime (Fortaz, Tazidime), cefoperazone (Cefobid), or cefepime (Maxipime), a fourth-generation cephalosporin, have predictable activity against P aeruginosa. Ceftazidime has greater activity than cefoperazone and is the one used most often in veterinary medicine. Cefoperazone is no longer marketed.

Cefpodoxime and Cefovecin

Cefpodoxime is more active than many other third-generation cephalosporins against Staphylococcus, and pharmacokinetic properties allow once-daily dosing.[28] However, it is not active against P aeruginosa, Enterococcus, or methicillin-resistant Staphylococcus. Examination of wild-type distributions[29] also indicates that it is not a true third-generation cephalosporin in terms of activity against Enterobacteriaceae (for example E coli). The minimum inhibition concentration (MIC) for cefpodoxime is 8-fold higher than that for cefotaxime and 4-fold higher than that for ceftazidime against wild-type strains of E coli (wild-type cutoff values).

In the spring of 2008, cefovecin (Convenia) was registered by the US Food and Drug Administration (FDA) Center for Veterinary Medicine for use in dogs and cats for treatment of routine skin infections, and previously had been approved in other countries for routine skin infections and urinary tract infections. There have been pharmacokinetic studies published for dogs and cats,[30,31] pharmacodynamic studies published,[32] and clinical efficacy studies in dogs and cats.[33–36] In the clinical studies, cefovecin was compared with another active antimicrobial (cefadroxil, cephalexin, or amoxicillin-clavulanate) and was noninferior to these other drugs.

There are currently no CLSI-approved standards for susceptibility testing established for cefovecin.[1] Based on the distribution of organisms reported,[32] less than or equal to 2.0 μg/mL should be considered for a susceptible breakpoint. It has acceptable activity against wild-type strains of Staphylococcus species and gram-negative bacteria of the Enterobacteriaceae (eg, E coli, Klebsiella). However, activity against P aeruginosa is poor and it is not effective against methicillin-resistant staphylococci.

Even though cefovecin is classified as a third-generation cephalosporin based on structure, it is not as active against gram-negative bacteria as the other third-generation cephalosporins. It should not be regarded as a drug to use for bacteria that have already shown resistance to other agents. Although it had greater activity against gram-negative bacteria, as demonstrated by the MIC_{90} (MIC required to inhibit the growth of 90% of organisms) values of 1 μg/mL, compared with 16 μg/mL for cephalexin and cefadroxil,[36] other third-generation cephalosporins (eg, ceftazidime, cefotaxime) are more active and have lower MIC values. Moreover, the free (protein unbound) plasma concentrations of cefovecin are not sustained highly enough throughout the dose interval to be considered for treatment of systemic infections against gram-negative bacilli.

Based on these observations, although cefovecin and cefpodoxime are technically considered third-generation cephalosporins, the activities of cephalosporins within these arbitrary generations are not always similar. Cefovecin and cefpodoxime are not as active against gram-negative bacteria as injectable third-generation cephalosporins used in human medicine, such as ceftazidime or cefotaxime.

Carbapenems

The β-lactam antibiotics with greatest activity against *P aeruginosa* are the carbapenems. The carbapenems are β-lactam antibiotics that include imipenem-cilastatin sodium (Primaxin), meropenem (Merrem), ertapenem (Invanz), and, most recently, doripenem (Doribax). All drugs in this group have activity against the enteric gram-negative bacilli. Ertapenem does not have anti-*Pseudomonas* activity. Resistance (carbapenemases) among veterinary isolates has been rare. Imipenem is administered with cilastatin to decrease renal tubular metabolism. Imipenem has become a valuable antibiotic because it has a broad spectrum that includes many bacteria resistant to other drugs. Imipenem is not active against methicillin-resistant staphylococci or resistant strains of *E faecium*. The high activity of imipenem is attributed to its stability against most of the β-lactamases (including extended spectrum β-lactamase) and ability to penetrate porin channels that usually exclude other drugs.[37] The carbapenems are more rapidly bactericidal than the cephalosporins and less likely to induce release of endotoxin in an animal from gram-negative sepsis.

Some disadvantages of imipenem are the inconvenience of administration, short shelf life after reconstitution, and high cost. It must be diluted in fluids before administration. Meropenem, a more recent carbapenem (some experts consider it a second-generation penem) and has antibacterial activity greater than imipenem against some isolates. One important advantage compared with imipenem is that it is more soluble and can be administered in a smaller fluid volume and more rapidly. For example, small volumes can be administered subcutaneously with almost complete absorption. There also is a lower incidence of adverse effects to the central nervous system, such as seizures. Based on pharmacokinetic experiments in our laboratory,[38] the recommended dose for Enterobacteriaceae and other sensitive organisms is 8.5 mg/kg SC every 12 hours, or 24 mg/kg IV every 12 hours. For infections caused by *P aeruginosa* or other similar organisms that may have MIC values as high as 1.0 μg/mL, the dose is 12 mg/kg every 8 hours, SC, or 25 mg/kg every 8 hours, IV. For susceptible organisms in the urinary tract, 8 mg/kg, SC, every 12 hours can be used. In our experience, these doses have been well tolerated except for slight hair loss over some of the SC dosing sites.

Penicillins

Penicillin derivatives with activity against *P aeruginosa* and the Enterobacteriaceae include the ureidopenicillins (mezlocillin, azlocillin, piperacillin) and the carboxylic derivatives of penicillin (carbenicillin, ticarcillin). These derivatives are available as sodium salts for injection; there are no orally effective formulations in this class, except indanyl carbenicillin (Geocillin, Geopen), which is poorly absorbed and not useful for systemic infections. These drugs are more expensive than the more commonly used penicillins, and must be administered frequently (eg, at least 4 times daily in patients with normal kidney function) to be effective. Dosage regimens for these drugs have been published in other sources.[25,26] Ticarcillin is usually administered in combination with the β-lactamase inhibitor clavulanic acid (Timentin). Because these drugs degrade quickly after reconstitution, observe the storage recommendations on the package insert to preserve the drug's potency.

Fluoroquinolones

Once a resistant strain of the Enterobacteriaceae (eg, *E coli, Klebsiella pneumoniae*) has been identified, the fluoroquinolones are rarely an available choice for treatment.[39] These strains are usually multidrug resistant and susceptibility to fluoroquinolones is unlikely. In addition, fluoroquinolone activity may be especially unpredictable if the patient has previously been treated with this class of agents. Previous exposure to fluoroquinolones may select for resistant strains of *E coli* in dogs that can persist long after drug treatment has been discontinued.[40]

In some cases, a fluoroquinolone may be active against *P aeruginosa*. When administering a fluoroquinolone to treat *P aeruginosa*, the high end of the dose range is suggested because even among wild-type strains the MIC values are higher than for other gram-negative bacteria. Of the currently available fluoroquinolones (human or veterinary), ciprofloxacin is the most active against *P aeruginosa*, followed by marbofloxacin, enrofloxacin, difloxacin, and orbifloxacin.[41,42] Note that this ranking applies to in vitro activity (comparison of MIC values) and does not attempt to predict the comparative efficacy of these drugs. Ciprofloxacin oral absorption can be unpredictable in dogs and there is no assurance that effective concentrations will be achieved after oral administration.[43] Ciprofloxacin is poorly absorbed from oral administration in cats and is not expected to attain effective concentrations.[44]

Aminoglycosides

Aminoglycosides are active against most wild-type strains of *P aeruginosa*. Against resistant isolates, amikacin and tobramycin are more active than gentamicin, and resistance is less likely to these drugs.[7] When availability of amikacin has been limited, veterinarians have used tobramycin as an alternative. Aminoglycosides are valuable for treating gram-negative bacilli that are resistant to other drugs. They are rapidly bactericidal, less expensive than the injectable drugs listed earlier, and can be administered once daily. Among these, amikacin and tobramycin are the most active and the first choice in small animal medicine when resistant or refractory infections are encountered. Both drugs can be administered once daily IV, IM, or SC.

There are 3 disadvantages to systemic use of aminoglycosides[45]: (1) when treatment must extend for 2 weeks or longer, the risk of kidney injury is greater with longer duration of treatment. (2) They must be injected (except for topical uses), which some pet owners are reluctant to perform. (3) Activity of aminoglycosides is diminished in the presence of pus and cellular debris,[46] which may decrease their usefulness for the treatment of wound and ear infections that are characterized by this environment, such as infections caused by *P aeruginosa*. Strategies to decrease the risk of drug-induced kidney injury from aminoglycosides are discussed later in this article.

DRUG CHOICES FOR METHICILLIN-RESISTANT *STAPHYLOCOCCUS* AND RESISTANT *ENTEROCOCCUS* SPECIES

Because susceptibility to non–β-lactam antibiotics is unpredictable, a susceptibility test is needed to identify the most appropriate drug to administer for these infections. Chloramphenicol, tetracyclines, aminoglycosides (gentamicin, amikacin), and rifampin are drugs to consider for these infections if a susceptibility test can confirm activity. These drugs are discussed in more detail elswhere[27] and briefly later in this article. Unlike the human strains of community-acquired *S aureus*, the veterinary strains of MRSP are usually not susceptible to trimethoprim-sulfonamides, clindamycin, or fluoroquinolones.[17,47] However, a susceptibility test should always be used to confirm whether or not these drugs may have activity against isolates from animals. The use of these medications in veterinary dermatology has been discussed previously.[48–50] Most staphylococci are also susceptible to nitrofurantoin, but this drug is used only for urinary tract infections. Topical drugs also should be considered for treatment of localized infections. These drugs (eg, mupirocin or fusidic acid) are available in topical ointments and have been used in dogs and cats.

Rifampin (Rifampicin)

Rifampin, also known in some countries as rifampicin, is an old antibiotic that has seen recent interest because of its activity against methicillin-resistant *Staphylococcus*. Equine practitioners have been familiar with rifampin for many years because of its use for treating infections caused by *Rhodococcus equi*. Small animal veterinarians are now being introduced to this antibiotic because of its activity against methicillin-resistant *Staphylococcus*. This antibiotic may be new to small animal veterinarians, but was originally discovered in the pine forests of France in the 1950s and was introduced into clinical medicine in the 1960s. Rifampin is the United States Pharmacopeia official name, and rifampicin is the International Nonproprietary Name and British Approved Name; the names are synonymous. Rifamycin and rifabutin are structurally similar antibiotics(they are in the group of rifamycins) but they are not identical.

Rifampin is a bactericidal antibiotic that acts by inhibiting bacterial RNA polymerase. It is highly lipophilic, with a high volume of distribution and good absorption in most animal species studied. The intracellular penetration has made this drug valuable for treating intracellular bacteria in people and animals, including *Mycobacterium* and *R equi*. Rifampin is active against most strains of MRSP,[47] although resistance among canine isolates has been identified.[51] Rifampin has been effective for treatment of canine pyoderma caused by *S pseudintermedius* at a dose of 5 mg/kg once daily for 10 days.[52] A dose of 10 mg/kg per day, usually split into 2 doses 12 hours apart, has been recommended,[26,27] although some veterinary formularies have recommend a much higher dose.

Resistance occurs through mutations and clonal spread of a resistant strain. To reduce the rate of mutation, combination therapy with other agents has usually been recommended in human guidelines,[53] as was the recommendation from a veterinary study.[51] However, experimental infections caused by *Staphylococcus* have been successfully treated with rifampin monotherapy.[54] In a review of the evidence from clinical trials of eradication of *S aureus* in humans, rifampin was also an effective agent for eradication of *S aureus*, whether administered as monotherapy or as a combination.[53] Addition of a second antibiotic did not seem to confer additional effectiveness to rifampin monotherapy for eradication of methicillin-resistant *Staphylococcus*. As the investigators pointed out, "...the decrease in the development of resistance to rifampin with the use of combination therapy has been mainly validated in clinical situations in which long-term therapy with rifampin was necessary (eg, tuberculosis) and may not be the same for short-term treatment for *S aureus* carriage eradication."

Interactions and adverse effects

Rifampin is a strong inducer of drug metabolizing enzymes. According to one article, "The list of drugs that interact with rifampin is remarkably long."[55] Induction can significantly increase the metabolism and clearance of other coadministered drugs that are affected by these proteins. The consequence of induction is diminished effect of the coadministered drug and it may require a higher dose or more frequent administration. For example, rifampin coadministration significantly affects the exposure to prednisolone.[56] In people, 4 weeks are required for full recovery of the rifampin effect after discontinuation.[54,55] Rifamin may also have dual effects in which it can be an inhibitor of intestinal transport as well as an inducer of other proteins.

Adverse effects, which are associated with high doses, include liver injury and gastrointestinal disturbance. In dogs, hepatotoxicosis is the most common adverse reaction and 20% to 26% of dogs receiving 5 to 10 mg/kg develop increases in liver enzymes, and some develop hepatitis. Dogs seem to be more susceptible to liver injury than humans. To avoid adverse effects, it is recommended not to exceed a dose of 10 mg/kg per day and periodically monitor liver enzymes. Rifampin has an unpalatable taste. It also may produce a discoloration (orange-red color) to the urine, tears, and sclera. Owners should be warned of this possibility.

Tetracyclines (Doxycycline, Minocycline)

Some MRSP are susceptible to tetracyclines. Because the choice of oral tetracyclines is limited for small animals, either doxycycline or minocycline should be used. Both are at least as active, and perhaps more active in vitro, against *Staphylococcus* species.

Doxycycline

Doxycycline administration to small animals is usually accomplished with tablets (50, 75, 100 mg) or oral suspension (5 mg/mL suspension and 10 mg/mL syrup) at doses of 5 mg/kg twice daily. When compounded in a suspension in a more concentrated form (either 33.3 mg/mL or 167 mg/mL) in an aqueous-based vehicle, the formulation was stable for 7 days, but declined to only 20% of the initial potency at 14 days.[57]

Adverse effects from doxycycline have been rare. Renal injury, intestinal disturbances, or hepatic injury is uncommon. Unlike other tetracyclines, it has little affinity for calcium and does not cause the dental enamel discoloration known for other tetracyclines, and does not chelate with calcium-containing oral products. Its oral absorption is not affected by administration of sucralfate, compared to other tetracyclines. It has been mixed with chocolate milk for administration to children with no interference with absorption.

An adverse reaction associated with doxycycline hyclate is injury to the esophagus from a broken tablet or incompletely dissolved capsule. This reaction has been documented in cats and is probably the result of the hydrochloride (HCl) contact with the esophageal mucosal owing to slow transit through the esophagus. This problem has been primarily associated with doxycycline hyclate (the form most common in the United States), rather than doxycycline monohydrate.

This reaction can be alleviated by administration of oral doxycycline hyclate with a water flush or immediate feeding to ensure that the medication passes to the stomach.

Minocycline

Minocycline can be considered as an alternative if doxycycline is not available. Minocycline is at least as active against bacteria as other tetracyclines. There has been not been as much clinical experience with minocycline as with doxycycline; however, it may be acceptable when other alternatives are not available.

Only limited susceptibility data for minocycline are available, but it is likely that some isolates of MRSP may be susceptible to minocycline even though they are resistant to other tetracyclines. It depends on whether or not the bacteria carries the tet(M) resistance or just the tet(K) resistance. *Staphylococcus* strains that are tetracycline resistant because of efflux mediated by *tet*(K) may still be susceptible to minocycline; however, resistance caused by the ribosomal protection mechanism *tet*(M) produces cross-resistance to both doxycycline and minocycline. Published data so far on activity of minocycline against resistant strains from animals[58] and some other preliminary data are encouraging.

In humans, minocycline is rapidly and almost completely absorbed after oral administration. In people, it is 75% protein bound, has a volume of distribution (V_d) of 1.17 L/kg and has a half-life ($t_{1/2}$) of 15 to 19 hours. Between 5% and 12% of the minocycline dose is recovered in urine. Details of the oral pharmacokinetics have not been reported for dogs. Protein binding is reported to be 75% in dogs,[59] which is lower than for doxycycline, but this value was from an unreferenced source, and more recent studies indicate that protein binding in dogs may be only 50–60%. From the published study of IV minocycline in dogs,[60] it had a terminal half-life of approximately 7 hours, which is less than half of the value reported for people. The V_d was greater than 2 L/kg in dogs, which is almost twice that of people. Both of these values suggest that extrapolation of doses from people is likely to be ineffective.

The extent of oral absorption in dogs or cats is not known. In people it is almost complete. However, if oral absorption is calculated based on area-under-the-curve (AUC) values provided in a previous study,[61] it suggests a much lower oral absorption rate in dogs than in people: only 20%. Only 2.2% of the oral dose was excreted in the urine. Minocycline seems to be safe in dogs. In the previously cited study,[61] dogs tolerated 30 mg/kg per day for 30 days, and did not see adverse effects until doses were increased to 40 mg/kg. However, there are anecdotal accounts of gastrointestinal upset from minocycline in dogs at therapeutic doses.

Because of the shortage of data on minocycline, the most effective dose is not known. But if 1 the V_d, protein binding, half-life, clearance, and AUC/MIC target are considered, an approximate dose is 5–10 mg/kg every 12 hours.

For either doxycycline or minocycline, the current CLSI breakpoint to determine susceptibility is not recommended.[1] The doxycycline breakpoint for humans is less than or equal to 4 μg/mL, which is probably too high for dogs. It is likely much lower, and less than or equal to 0.12 μg/mL is more reasonable based on MIC distributions and pharmacokinetic/pharmacodynamic (PK/PD) data. The equivalent breakpoint for susceptible bacteria if tetracycline is used for testing is less than or equal to 0.5 μg/mL. It is difficult to attain the AUC/MIC target using a breakpoint of 4 μg/mL; a lower breakpoint is recommended. CLSI may consider a veterinary-specific breakpoint at a later time.

Chloramphenicol

Chloramphenicol was popular decades ago, but its use diminished in the 1970s and 1980s because other active and safer drugs became available. The small animal formulation is approved by the FDA (Chloromycetin) but is not actively marketed. Chloramphenicol has the disadvantage of a narrow margin of safety in dogs and cats, and the necessity of frequent administration in dogs to maintain adequate concentrations (3 or 4 times daily oral administration). These disadvantages still exist, but the activity of chloramphenicol against bacteria (eg, staphylococci and enterococci) that are resistant to other oral drugs has created increased use of chloramphenicol in recent years. Florfenicol (Nuflor), an injectable alternative for cattle and pigs, is cleared so rapidly in dogs that frequent high doses are necessary. There is no oral formulation of florfenicol for dogs and effective clinical doses have not been established.

Chloramphenicol has FDA approval for use in dogs as 100, 250, and 500 mg tablets (Chloromycetin). The oral suspension of chloramphenicol palmitate is rarely available. Although chloramphenicol is poorly soluble (<5 mg/mL), the poor solubility does not interfere with oral absorption. Chloramphenicol is absorbed orally with or without food (except some formulations in cats). Tablets and capsules have similar oral absorption in dogs.

Dose recommendations

Plasma concentrations of chloramphenicol were published in several studies and summarized in a review.[27] Using Monte Carlo simulations and available pharmacokinetic parameters, a dose of 50 mg/kg by mouth to dogs, every 8 hours attains antibacterial concentrations greater than the MIC value of 8 μg/mL in most animals. There is some evidence that chloramphenicol may be more bactericidal against *Staphylococcus* than previously thought.

Adverse effects and interactions

Significant disadvantages of chloramphenicol are adverse effects and drug interactions. As cited earlier, chloramphenicol has a narrow margin of safety. The recommend dose of 50 mg/kg every 8 hours in dogs frequently produces gastrointestinal problems. High doses easily produce toxicity in dogs.[62] A decrease in protein synthesis in the bone marrow may be associated with chronic treatment. This effect is most prominent in cats, but can occur in any animals. Idiosyncratic aplastic anemia is possible from exposure to people, but has not been described in animals. The incidence of aplastic anemia is rare but the consequences are severe because it is irreversible. Because exposure to humans can potentially produce severe consequences, veterinarians should caution pet owners about handling the medications, and to ensure that accidental human exposure does not occur at home.

Chloramphenicol is notorious for producing drug interactions. Chloramphenicol is an inhibitor of cytochrome P450 CYP2B11, and possibly other enzymes, in dogs.[63,64] Therefore, chloramphenicol can decrease the clearance of other drugs that are metabolized by the same metabolic enzymes. Chloramphenicol inhibits the metabolism of opiates, barbiturates, propofol, phenytoin, salicylate, and perhaps other drugs.[64–67]

A previously unrecognized problem is the association between chloramphenicol administration and neurologic problems in dogs. In some dogs (some anecdotal accounts indicate that large breeds are more susceptible) reversible neurologic deficits are possible, which manifest as paresis, ataxia, and hind limb dysfunction. The mechanism for this reaction is unknown.

Aminoglycosides (Gentamicin, Amikacin)

Aminoglycosides (specifically amikacin and gentamicin) have consistent in vitro activity against *Staphylococcus*, including methicillin-resistant strains of *S pseudintermedius*. The disadvantages of aminoglycosides were discussed earlier in this article. Because oral absorption is not possible, these agents must be administered by injection and there is a potential for kidney injury in animals from prolonged use. The risk of kidney injury is higher if animals have prior evidence of kidney disease.[45]

Aminoglycosides are rapidly bactericidal and can be administered once daily.[68] In hospital, the route is usually IV, but dog and cat owners have been trained to administer SC or IM injections at home. Because these are water-soluble formulations, they are well absorbed from SC and IM injection sites, although these routes may produce pain in some patients. Gentamicin also is a component of many topical formulations used for skin infections.

For gentamicin, the current CLSI breakpoint for susceptible bacteria[1] is less than or equal to 2 μg/mL for gram-negative bacteria (assuming a dose of 10 mg/kg every 24 hours), but these values are probably appropriate for *Staphylococcus* species as well. There is no veterinary-specific breakpoint for amikacin. The human CLSI susceptibility breakpoint for amikacin is less than or equal to 16 μg/mL,[1] but most veterinary isolates are probably less than or equal to 4 µg/mL. Activity of aminoglycosides is diminished in the presence of pus and cellular debris,[46] which may be important for some skin infections. These conditions may decrease the usefulness for the treatment of wound and ear infections.

Although aminoglycosides have in vitro activity against *Staphylococcus* and *Enterococcus*, their clinical efficacy as single agents for treating infections caused by these organisms in animals has not been reported. These drugs are usually considered excellent bactericidal drugs for gram-negative bacilli, but clinical efficacy for gram-positive cocci is less certain. In addition to their effect on bacterial ribosomes, an additional (and perhaps more important) mechanism is that these agents act to disrupt the cell surface biofilm, particularly on gram-negative bacteria, to produce disruption, loss of cell wall integrity, and a rapid bactericidal effect. This property is not as prominent for gram-positive bacteria and these drugs are not as active against gram-positive bacteria unless administered with a cell wall disrupting agent such as vancomycin or a β-lactam antibiotic.

Adverse effects

The most serious toxic effect associated with aminoglycoside therapy is kidney injury.[45] Toxicity initially affects the renal proximal tubules because of active uptake in these cells. The entire nephron can eventually be affected. Animals that are dehydrated, have electrolyte imbalances (for example low Na^+ or K^+), are septicemic, or have existing renal disease are at a higher risk for toxicity than healthy animals. Kidney injury is attributed to persistent drug levels (especially high trough concentrations) throughout the dose interval. Therefore, extended once-a-day dosing intervals decrease risk of kidney injury.[68]

Glycopeptides (Vancomycin)

Of the glycopeptides, vancomycin is the only one used in veterinary medicine. Although vancomycin is an old drug, it is unfamiliar to most veterinarians. It is difficult to administer to small animals because of the need to administer IV and the requirement for a slow infusion. Despite is long history of use in people, there are uncertainties and better alternatives are being sought.[69] Resistance to vancomycin among *S aureus* is rare, but MIC values may be shifting higher. Resistance among *S pseudintermedius* has not been reported. Vancomycin-resistant enterococci are an important problem in human medicine but are rare in veterinary medicine.

Dosing regimens

Vancomycin is bacteridical for staphylococci by inhibiting the cell wall in a time-dependent manner. Vancomycin is poorly absorbed orally and this route should not be used except to treat intestinal infections. IM administration is painful and irritating to tissues. The usual dosage for small animals is 15 mg/kg every 8 hours, IV, via slow infusion. Therapeutic drug monitoring can be performed to ensure that trough concentrations are maintained at more than 10 µg/mL for skin and soft tissue infections.

Adverse effects

If vancomycin is administered according to the recommended dosing rates, adverse reactions are rare. Early formulations of vancomycin were associated with a high incidence of adverse effects. Most of these effects resulted from rapid IV administration, which induced flushing of the skin, pruritus, tachycardia and other signs attributed to histamine release. Nephrotoxicity and ototoxicity also were reported. Newer formulations are safer because impurities have been removed.

Some New Drugs

In response to the emergence of resistant gram-positive bacteria in humans (primarily methicillin-resistant *Staphylococcus* and drug-resistant *Enterococcus* spp), the pharmaceutical industry has responded with new antibiotics for people, but there has not been a similar response for treating resistant infections in animals. These drugs are generally expensive, and most of them must be administered by the IV route, in some cases via a central vein. They have primarily a gram-positive spectrum, but in some instances can be used for bacteria other than *Staphylococcus* or *Enterococcus*. Because of the expense, or the difficult administration, the use of these drugs has not been described in clinical veterinary patients. These drugs include streptogramins (combination of 30:70 quinupristin/dalfopristin, called Synercid); daptomycin (Cubicin), a cyclic lipopeptide antibiotic; telavancin, another glycopeptide; tigecycline (Tygacil), a unique tetracycline; linezolid (Zyvox), the first in the class of oxazolidinones; telithromycin (Ketek), the first of a class of drugs called ketolides (currently restricted because of toxicity risk in humans); and a new generation of cephalosporins, ceftaroline fosamil (Teflaro) and ceftobiprole. The only one of these agents that has been used in veterinary patients, to the author's knowledge, is linezolid, which is discussed briefly below.

Oxazolidinones

Linezolid (Zyvox) is the first in the class of oxazolidinones to be used in human medicine. There are no veterinary drugs in this class. It is used in people to treat methicillin-resistant *Staphylococcus* and vancomycin-resistant gram-positive infections caused by enterococci and streptococci. It has excellent activity against staphylococci and enterococci. Resistance has been documented,[70] but several sequential mutations are needed for development of resistance because of the redundant nature of the 23S rRNA gene, which codes for the target of this drug.

Pharmacokinetics and dosing
Linezolid is absorbed orally and also can be administered intravenously. Oral absorption is practically 100% in all animals tested,[71] and is not affected by food. Linezolid is metabolized similarly across species[71] and pharmacokinetic parameters scale allometrically across species, allowing accurate prediction of doses for both dogs and cats of approximately 10 mg/kg twice daily.[72]

Clinical use in animals
Because of the high expense, linezolid has been used infrequently in veterinary medicine, and probably will remain a rarely used medication. Its use at this time has only been reported in unpublished anecdotal canine and feline cases, which have responded with good outcomes.

Adverse effects
Toxicokinetic studies in dogs at high doses showed that linezolid was well tolerated and did not accumulate.[71] Linezolid is a mild, reversible inhibitor on monoamine oxidases A and B. In the 10 years of clinical use of linezolid in people, these theoretic interactions with adrenergic agents have not been significant. Whether or not linezolid will produce interactions in dogs administered adrenergic agents (eg, phenylpropanolamine, selegiline) or other drugs metabolized by monoamine oxidases (eg, serotonin reuptake inhibitors or tricyclic antidepressants) has not been studied. Long-term use (>14 days) can cause bone marrow suppression (eg, thrombocytopenia) in people, but this has not been reported in dogs or cats. If it occurs, myelosuppression is mild and reversible.

REFERENCES

1. Clinical Laboratory Standards Institute (CLSI). Performance standards for antimicrobial disk and dilution susceptibility tests for bacteria isolated from animals. Approved Standard. 3rd edition. Wayne (PA): Clinical and Laboratory Standards Institute; 2008. CLSI document M31–A3.
2. Oluoch AO, Kim CH, Weisiger RM, et al. Nonenteric *Escherichia coli* isolates from dogs: 674 cases (1990-1998). J Am Vet Med Assoc 2001;218:381–4.
3. Torres SM, Diaz SF, Nogueira SA, et al. Frequency of urinary tract infection among dogs with pruritic disorders receiving long-term glucocorticoid treatment. J Am Vet Med Assoc 2005;227:239–43.
4. Shaheen BW, Boothe DM, Oyarzabal OA, et al. Antimicrobial resistance profiles and clonal relatedness of canine and feline *Escherichia coli* pathogens expressing multidrug resistance in the United States. J Vet Intern Med 2010;24: 323–30.
5. Martin Barrasa JL, Lupiola Gomez P, Gonzalez Lama Z, et al. Antibacterial susceptibility patterns of *Pseudomonas* strains isolated from chronic canine otitis externa. J Vet Med B Infect Dis Vet Public Health 2000;47:191–6.
6. Colombini S, Merchant RS, Hosgood G. Microbial flora and antimicrobial susceptibility patterns from dogs with otitis media. Vet Dermatol 2000;11: 235–9.
7. Petersen AD, Walker RD, Bowman MM, et al. Frequency of isolation and antimicrobial susceptibility patterns of *Staphylococcus intermedius* and *Pseudomonas aeruginosa* isolates from canine skin and ear samples over a 6 year period (1992-1997). J Am Anim Hosp Assoc 2002;38:407–13.
8. Pinchbeck LR, Cole LK, Hillier A, et al. Pulsed-field gel electrophoresis patterns and antimicrobial susceptibility phenotypes for coagulase-positive staphylococcal isolates from pustules and carriage sites in dogs with superficial bacterial folliculitis. Am J Vet Res 2007;68(5):535–42.
9. Lloyd DH, Lamport AI, Feeney C. Sensitivity to antibiotics amongst cutaneous and mucosal isolates of canine pathogenic staphylococci in the UK, 1980-1996. Vet Dermatol 1996;7:171–5.
10. Bond R, Loeffler A. What's happened to *Staphylococcus intermedius*? Taxonomic revision and emergence of multi-drug resistance. J Small Anim Pract 2012;53:147–54.
11. Weese JS, van Duijkeren E. Methicillin-resistant *Staphylococcus aureus* and *Staphylococcus pseudintermedius* in veterinary medicine. Vet Microbiol 2010; 140(3–4):418–29.
12. Weese JS. Methicillin-resistant *Staphylococcus aureus*: an emerging pathogen in small animals. J Am Anim Hosp Assoc 2005;41(3):150–7.
13. Gortel K, Campbell KL, Kakoma I, et al. Methicillin resistance among staphylococci isolated from dogs. Am J Vet Res 1999;60:1526–30.
14. Deresinski S. Methicillin-resistant *Staphylococcus aureus*: an evolutionary, epidemiologic, and therapeutic odyssey. Clin Infect Dis 2005;40:562–73.
15. Jones RD, Kania SA, Rohrbach BW, et al. Prevalence of oxacillin- and multidrug-resistant staphylococci in clinical samples from dogs: 1,772 samples (2001-2005). J Am Vet Med Assoc 2007;230(2):221–7.
16. Bemis DA, Jones RD, Hiatt LE, et al. Comparison of tests to detect oxacillin resistance in *Staphylococcus intermedius*, *Staphylococcus schleiferi*, and *Staphylococcus aureus* isolates from canine hosts. J Clin Microbiol 2006; 44(9):3374–6.

17. Bemis DA, Jones RD, Frank LA, et al. Evaluation of susceptibility test break-points used to predict mecA-mediated resistance in *Staphylococcus pseudintermedius* isolated from dogs. J Vet Diagn Invest 2009;21(1):53–8.
18. Sasaki T, Kikuchi K, Tanaka Y, et al. Reclassification of phenotypically identified *Staphylococcus intermedius* strains. J Clin Microbiol 2007;45:2770–8.
19. Bannoehr J, Guardabassi L. *Staphylococcus pseudintermedius* in the dog: taxonomy, diagnostics, ecology, epidemiology and pathogenicity. Vet Dermatol 2012;23:253–66.
20. Dancer SJ. The effect of antibiotics on methicillin-resistant *Staphylococcus aureus*. J Antimicrob Chemother 2008;61:246–53.
21. Harbarth S, Samore MH. Interventions to control MRSA: high time for time-series analysis? J Antimicrob Chemother 2008;62:431–3.
22. Paterson DL. "Collateral damage" from cephalosporin or quinolone antibiotic therapy. Clin Infect Dis 2004;38(Suppl 4):S341–5.
23. Prescott JF, Hanna WJ, Reid-Smith R, et al. Antimicrobial drug use and resistance in dogs. Can Vet J 2002;43:107–16.
24. Bartlett JG. Intra-abdominal sepsis. Med Clin North Am 1995;79(3):599–617.
25. Papich MG. Handbook of antimicrobial therapy for small animals. St Louis (MO): Elsevier-Saunders; 2011. p. 140.
26. Papich MG. Saunders handbook of veterinary drugs. 3rd edition. St Louis (MO): Elsevier-Saunders; 2011. p. 858.
27. Papich MG. Selection of antibiotics for methicillin-resistant *Staphylococcus pseudintermedius*: time to revisit some old drugs? Vet Dermatol 2012;23(4): 352–60.
28. Papich MG, Davis JL, Floerchinger AM. Pharmacokinetics, protein binding, and tissue distribution of orally administered cefpodoxime proxetil and cephalexin in dogs. Am J Vet Res 2010;71(12):1484–91.
29. Available at: http://www.eucast.org/mic_distributions/. Accessed May 26, 2013.
30. Stegemann MR, Sherington J, Blanchflower S. Pharmacokinetics and pharmacodynamics of cefovecin in dogs. J Vet Pharmacol Ther 2006;29(6):501–11. PMID: 17083454.
31. Stegemann MR, Sherington J, Coati N, et al. Pharmacokinetics of cefovecin in cats. J Vet Pharmacol Ther 2006;29(6):513–24. PMID: 17083455.
32. Stegemann MR, Passmore CA, Sherington J, et al. Antimicrobial activity and spectrum of cefovecin, a new extended-spectrum cephalosporin, against pathogens collected from dogs and cats in Europe and North America. Antimicrob Agents Chemother 2006;50(7):2286–92. PMID: 16801403.
33. Stegemann MR, Coati N, Passmore CA, et al. Clinical efficacy and safety of cefovecin in the treatment of canine pyoderma and wound infections. J Small Anim Pract 2007;48(7):378–86. PMID: 17559523.
34. Stegemann MR, Sherington J, Passmore C. The efficacy and safety of cefovecin in the treatment of feline abscesses and infected wounds. J Small Anim Pract 2007;48(12):683–9. PMID: 17725587.
35. Passmore CA, Sherington J, Stegemann MR. Efficacy and safety of cefovecin (Convenia) for the treatment of urinary tract infections in dogs. J Small Anim Pract 2007;48(3):139–44. PMID: 17355604.
36. Six R, Cherni J, Chesebrough R, et al. Efficacy and safety of cefovecin in treating bacterial folliculitis, abscesses, or infected wounds in dogs. J Am Vet Med Assoc 2008;233(3):433–9.
37. Livermore DM. Of *Pseudomonas*, porins, pumps, and carbapenems. J Antimicrob Chemother 2001;47:247–50.

38. Bidgood T, Papich MG. Plasma pharmacokinetics and tissue fluid concentrations of meropenem after intravenous and subcutaneous administration in dogs. Am J Vet Res 2002;63(12):1622–8.
39. Papich MG, Riviere JE. Chapter 38. Fluoroquinolone antimicrobial drugs. In: Riviere JE, Papich MG, editors. Veterinary pharmacology and therapeutics. 9th edition. Ames (IA): Wiley-Blackwell Publishing; 2009. p. 1524.
40. Boothe DM, Debavalya N. Impact of routine antimicrobial therapy on canine fecal *Escherichia coli* antimicrobial resistance: a pilot study. Int J Appl Res Vet Med 2011;9(4):396–406.
41. Riddle C, Lemons C, Papich MG, et al. Evaluation of ciprofloxacin as a representative of veterinary fluoroquinolones in susceptibility testing. J Clin Microbiol 2000;38:1636–7.
42. Rubin J, Walker RD, Blickenstaff K, et al. Antimicrobial resistance and genetic characterization of fluoroquinolone resistance of *Pseudomonas aeruginosa* isolated from canine infections. Vet Microbiol 2008;131(1–2):164–72.
43. Papich MG. Ciprofloxacin pharmacokinetics and oral absorption of generic ciprofloxacin tablets in dogs. Am J Vet Res 2012;73(7):1085–91.
44. Albarellos GA, Kreil VE, Landoni MF. Pharmacokinetics of ciprofloxacin after single intravenous and repeat oral administration to cats. J Vet Pharmacol Ther 2004;27:155–62.
45. Papich MG, Riviere JE. Chapter 36. Aminoglycoside antibiotics. In: Riviere JE, Papich MG, editors. Veterinary pharmacology and therapeutics. 9th edition. Ames (IA): Wiley-Blackwell Publishing; 2009. p. 1524.
46. Konig C, Simmen HP, Blaser J. Bacterial concentrations in pus and infected peritoneal fluid – implication of bactericidal activity of antibiotics. J Antimicrob Chemother 1998;42:227–32.
47. Perreten V, Kadlec K, Schwarz S, et al. Clonal spread of methicillin-resistant *Staphylococcus pseudintermedius* in Europe and North America: an international multicentre study. J Antimicrob Chemother 2010;65:1137–44.
48. Ihrke PJ, Papich MG, DeManuelle TC. The use of fluoroquinolones in veterinary dermatology. Vet Dermatol 1999;10:193–204.
49. Campbell KL. Sulphonamides: updates on use in veterinary medicine. Vet Dermatol 1999;10:205–15.
50. Noli C, Boothe D. Macrolides and lincosamides. Vet Dermatol 1999;10:217–23.
51. Kadlec K, van Duijkeren E, Wagenaar JA, et al. Molecular basis of rifampicin resistance in methicillin-resistant *Staphylococcus pseudintermedius* isolates from dogs. J Antimicrob Chemother 2011;66:1236–42.
52. Sentürk S, Özel E, Sen A. Clinical efficacy of rifampicin for treatment of canine pyoderma. Acta Vet Brno 2005;74:117–22.
53. Falagas ME, Bliziotis IA, Fragoulis KN. Oral rifampin for eradication of *Staphylococcus aureus* carriage from healthy and sick populations: a systematic review of the evidence from comparative trials. Am J Infect Control 2007; 35(2):106–14.
54. Lobo MC, Mandell GL. Treatment of experimental staphylococcal infection with rifampin. Antimicrob Agents Chemother 1972;2(3):195–200.
55. Reitman ML, Chu X, Cai S, et al. Rifampin's acute inhibitory and chronic inductive drug interactions: experimental and model-based approaches to drug-drug interaction trial design. Clin Pharmacol Ther 2011;89(2):234–42.
56. Lee KH, Shin JG, Chong WS, et al. Time course of the changes in prednisolone pharmacokinetics after co-administration or discontinuation of rifampin. Eur J Clin Pharmacol 1993;45(3):287–9.

57. Papich MG, Davidson GS, Fortier LA. Doxycycline concentration over time after storage in a compounded preparation for animals. J Am Vet Med Assoc 2013, in press.
58. Weese JS, Sweetman K, Edson H, et al. Evaluation of minocycline susceptibility of methicillin-resistant *Staphylococcus pseudintermedius*. Vet Microbiol 2013; 162(2–4):968–71.
59. Barza M, Brown RB, Shanks C, et al. Relation between lipophilicity and pharmacological behavior of minocycline, doxycycline, tetracycline, and oxytetracycline in dogs. Antimicrob Agents Chemother 1975;8(6):713–20.
60. Wilson RC, Kitzman JV, Kemp DT, et al. Compartmental and noncompartmental pharmacokinetic analyses of minocycline hydrochloride in the dog. Am J Vet Res 1985;46(6):1316–8.
61. Noble JF, Kanegis LA, Hallesy DW. Short-term toxicity and observations on certain aspects of the pharmacology of a unique tetracycline-minocycline. Toxicol Appl Pharmacol 1967;11(1):128–49.
62. Clark CH. Chloramphenicol dosage. Mod Vet Pract 1978;59(1):749–54.
63. Aidasani D, Zaya MJ, Malpas PB, et al. In vitro drug-drug interaction screens for canine veterinary medicines: evaluation of cytochrome P450 reversible inhibition. Drug Metab Dispos 2008;36:1512–8.
64. Kukanich B, Kukanich KS, Rodriguez JR. The effects of concurrent administration of cytochrome P-450 inhibitors on the pharmacokinetics of oral methadone in healthy dogs. Vet Anaesth Analg 2011;38(3):224–30.
65. Akesson CE, Linero PE. Effect of chloramphenicol on serum salicylate concentrations in dogs and cats. Am J Vet Res 1982;43:1471–2.
66. Sanders JE, Yoary RA, Fenner WR, et al. Interaction of phenytoin with chloramphenicol or pentobarbital in the dog. J Am Vet Med Assoc 1979;175(2):177–80.
67. Adams HR, Dixit BN. Prolongation of pentobarbital anesthesia by chloramphenicol in dogs and cats. J Am Vet Med Assoc 1970;156(7):902–5.
68. Drusano GL, Ambrose PG, Bhavnani SM, et al. Back to the future: using aminoglycosides again and how to dose them optimally. Clin Infect Dis 2007;45: 753–60.
69. Vandecasteele SJ, De Vriese AS, Tacconelli E. The pharmacokinetics and pharmacodynamics of vancomycin in clinical practice: evidence and uncertainties. J Antimicrob Chemother 2013;68:743–8.
70. Gu B, Kelesidis T, Tsiodras S, et al. The emerging problem of linezolid-resistant *Staphylococcus*. J Antimicrob Chemother 2013;68(1):4–11.
71. Slatter JG, Adams LA, Bush EC, et al. Pharmacokinetics, toxicokinetics, distribution, metabolism and excretion of linezolid in mouse, rat and dog. Xenobiotica 2002;32(10):907–24.
72. Bhamidipati RK, Dravid PV, Mullangi R, et al. Prediction of clinical pharmacokinetic parameters of linezolid using animal data by allometric scaling: applicability for the development of novel oxazolidinones. Xenobiotica 2004;36(6): 571–9.

Outpatient Oral Analgesics in Dogs and Cats Beyond Nonsteroidal Antiinflammatory Drugs: An Evidence-based Approach

Butch KuKanich, DVM, PhD

KEYWORDS

- Polysufated glycosaminoglycans • Amantadine • Tramadol • Gabapentin
- Pregabalin • Opioids • Antidepressants • Glucosamine

KEY POINTS

- Nonsteroidal antiinflammatory drugs are effective analgesics in dogs and cats, but adverse effects, preexisting conditions, and severity of pain may limit their use in some patients.
- Although many recommendations exist for additional analgesic use in dogs and cats, few of these recommendations are supported by controlled clinical trials.
- An injectable formulation of polysulfated glycosaminoglycans that is approved by the US Food and Drug Administration is an effective drug for controlling signs of arthritis in dogs, and amantadine in combination with meloxicam has shown efficacy in dogs with osteoarthritis.
- Oral tramadol was significantly better than placebo in controlling pain in dogs with arthritis, but the power of the study was low.
- Some data support further studies of gabapentin, pregabalin, hydrocodone, codeine, amitriptyline, and venlafaxine as analgesics in dogs and cats, but none of these drugs have shown efficacy in controlled clinical trials.
- Current data do not support the use of the oral opioids morphine, oxycodone, and methadone in dogs and cats because of low oral bioavailability.

INTRODUCTION

Treatment of outpatient pain in dogs and cats can be rewarding for the owners and veterinarians. Nonsteroidal antiinflammatory drugs (NSAIDs) are commonly administered to dogs and occasionally cats for controlling pain in an outpatient setting. There

Disclosures: the author has nothing to disclose.
Department of Anatomy and Physiology, Kansas State University, 228 Coles Hall, Manhattan, KS 66506, USA
E-mail address: kukanich@ksu.edu

are several NSAIDs approved by the US Food and Drug Administration (FDA) for dogs, with label indications of postoperative pain relief and management of osteoarthritis and there are a few that are FDA approved for cats for postoperative pain. Meloxicam is also approved by the European Medicines Agency for long-term control of musculoskeletal disorders in cats. Most animals tolerate NSAIDs well, with an expected 5% to 10% of patients having to discontinue treatment because of adverse effects, and up to 10% to 12% of patients potentially not responding to therapy. Adverse effects such as vomiting, diarrhea, gastrointestinal (GI) erosion/ulceration, nephropathy, or hepatopathy can occur. In addition, contraindications/precautions such as underlying renal disease, underlying hepatic disease, corticosteroid administration, or Cushing disease may preclude the use of NSAIDs. Therefore it is important to have knowledge of potential alternate therapeutics available and an understanding of the amount of information available supporting their use in dogs in cats (**Table 1**).

PHARMACOKINETICS AND THEIR APPLICATION TO ANALGESIC DOSAGE DESIGN

Pharmacokinetic studies are performed to describe the disposition of a drug in a particular species, after specific routes of administration, and at specific doses. Changes in route of administration, species, and dose can result in changes in the pharmacokinetic parameters. Therefore extrapolation of pharmacokinetic parameters to other species, routes of administration, or doses may not be accurate. In addition, many studies assess the pharmacokinetics of a drug after a single dose, but the pharmacokinetics may change with repeated doses, so extrapolating to multiple doses may not be accurate.[1,2]

Some drugs are metabolized to produce active metabolites that can contribute to the beneficial (and adverse) effects of the drug.[3] Some studies include the measurement and pharmacokinetics of active metabolites, but not all studies measure active metabolites and as such are incomplete descriptions of the potential factors contributing to the effects of the drugs.

Pharmacokinetic studies are useful in describing the extent and duration of drug exposure after an administered dose. Data derived from pharmacokinetic studies may be used to generate dose and interval recommendations to achieve and maintain desired concentrations, but that may not confer efficacy because there may be species-specific differences in the concentration or dose response to the drug. However, these recommendations are useful for designing experimental model studies, case studies, or controlled clinical trials.

Pharmacokinetic data are often used as a method of determining drug dosages. However, without corresponding data associating plasma concentrations with a clinical effect, the predictions may not be accurate because of differences in response to the drug. Pharmacokinetic studies provide a basis for potential effects or for dosages used in experimental study designs and controlled clinical trials.

Because many drugs are administered orally to dogs and cats, oral bioavailability is an important pharmacokinetic parameter. Oral bioavailability is the rate and extent of drug absorption after oral administration. However, bioavailability is often used to express only the fraction of dose absorbed, and it is used in that context in this article. High oral bioavailability implies that a large fraction of the dose is absorbed intact into systemic circulation after oral administration. Low oral bioavailability implies that a small fraction of the drug is absorbed.

Some factors affecting bioavailability include absorption of the drug from the site of administration (eg, a drug that is not absorbed has a low bioavailability), active efflux of the drug back into the lumen of the intestines after absorption, and presystemic

Table 1
Summary of drug characteristics for oral outpatient analgesia in dogs and cats

Drug	FDA Approved for Dogs or Cats?	Strength of Evidence	Relative Cost	Dose Frequency	DEA Scheduled	Other Notes
Polysulfated glycosaminoglycans	Yes, dogs	High	Moderate	Twice weekly	No	—
Amantadine	No	Moderate	Moderate	q 12–24 h	No	—
Tramadol	No	Low	Low	q 6–8 h	No[a]	Acetaminophen combinations toxic to cats
Gabapentin	No	Low	Low	q 8 h	No	—
Pregabalin	No	Low	High	q 12 h?	CV	—
Codeine	No	Low	Low	q 6–12 h	CII–CIII	Acetaminophen combinations toxic to cats
Hydrocodone	No	Low	Low	q 8–12 h	CIII	Acetaminophen combinations toxic to cats
Amitriptyline	No	Low	Low	q 12 h	No	—
Venlafaxine	No	Low	High	q 8–12 h	No	—
Duloxetine	No	None	High	—	No	—
Glucosamine and chondroitin	No	None	Moderate	q 24 h	No	—
Morphine	No	None	Low	—	CII	—
Oxycodone	No	None	Low	—	CII	Acetaminophen combinations toxic to cats
Methadone	No	None	Low	—	CII	—

Abbreviations: DEA, Drug Enforcement Agency; q, every.
[a] Some US states have restrictions on tramadol prescribing.

metabolism (metabolism of the drug after absorption, but before the drug entering systemic circulation). Codeine is a drug that is completely absorbed after oral administration to dogs, but only 4% of the parent drug reaches systemic circulation as codeine; the remaining 96% enters the systemic circulation as the active metabolite, codeine-6-glucuronide.[4] Therefore, despite complete codeine absorption in the dog, the oral bioavailability is only 4%.

Neither a high or low bioavailability absolutely predicts whether a drug can be effectively administered by a particular route. For example, diazepam has a low rectal bioavailability, but can be effective in controlling seizures in dogs because many active metabolites are formed during first-pass metabolism, producing a therapeutic effect.[5] In contrast, acetaminophen is well absorbed in dogs, with about a 50% oral bioavailability, but, because its elimination half-life is less than 1 hour, it requires a 4-hour (or shorter) dosing interval to maintain desired concentrations, which is not possible for many owners.[6]

Although low oral bioavailability can occasionally be overcome by increasing the drug dose, many times this is not an advisable strategy. Drugs with a low bioavailability also tend to have variable bioavailability, which makes dosing adjustments difficult. It is common for a drug with low oral bioavailability to have a 5-fold to 10-fold range in bioavailability, and the amount for any given animal on any given day can be within that range. Therefore selecting a dose with the intent to reach a desired plasma concentration can be difficult. For example, the oral bioavailability of meperidine ranged from 2% to 25% in 3 beagle dogs.[7] In addition, drugs may have dose-dependent changes in bioavailability caused by saturated absorption or metabolism pathways. Disproportional amounts of drug may be absorbed with changes in dose, which could produce drug toxicity. In contrast, less than proportional increases in the amount of drug absorbed can occur with increasing doses; for example, doubling the dose may only increase the total amount of drug absorbed from 4% to 5%.

CONTROLLED CLINICAL TRIALS

Controlled clinical trials are the best method of evaluating a drug for clinical use. The best study design for controlled clinical trials includes both positive and negative controls, has evaluators and administrators blinded to treatment to avoid bias, and randomly assigns animals to treatment groups to avoid bias. An excellent review of the design of clinical trials is available.[8]

Positive controls are needed to show that the study design can effectively determine the beneficial effects of the test treatment. For example, a study that includes only a negative control may generate a result of no significant difference between the test drug and the negative control. Without a positive control, it is not possible to determine whether the result is caused by a lack of effect of the test drug or by the evaluating method being unable to differentiate lack of benefit from a positive benefit. A negative control is needed to show that any measured benefit is the result of drug administration and not from observer bias or inability of the evaluation method to identify lack of an effect. Although a placebo effect is not typically thought of as occurring in animals, it has been documented and can be substantial: up to 25% (1 in 4 animals) as assessed by veterinarians and up to 39% (2 in 5 animals) as assessed by owners were reportedly improved on the Freedom of Information (FOI) summary for carprofen (New Animal Drug Application [NADA] 141-053). The percentage of responders in the placebo group, as evaluated by veterinarians, was 33% (1 in 3 animals) for the FOI for polysulfated glycosaminoglycans (NADA 141-038).

Some potential limitations of controlled clinical trials include that efficacy determined for one indication may not extrapolate to other disease conditions, the dose administered may not have been correct, the evaluating methods may not have been appropriate for the study, the study may not have had enough statistical power (sample size too small) to detect a true difference, the data may not be reproducible, and a perceived improvement was caused by random variability despite achieving a significant difference. Examples include that a drug effective for relieving osteoarthritis pain may not be effective for postoperative orthopedic pain and that the dose administered may have been too low and therefore lack of effect was only caused by lack of sufficient concentrations in the body.

Another major limitation of controlled clinical trials evaluating analgesics is that any method of evaluating efficacy is confounded by other factors. For example, pressure mat analysis, force plate, and lameness scores can be affected by gait independently of pain; owner questionnaires can have biased answers; and physiologic measurements can be affected by factors other than pain, such as stress of transport and evaluation. There is not currently a universally accepted measure of analgesia that is not confounded by other factors.

EXPERIMENTAL MODELS ASSESSING ANALGESICS IN ANIMALS

Experimental studies can be used to assess analgesic drugs. The most common types of models use thermal transducers (heat), mechanical stimulation (von Frey devices), electrical stimulation, or chemical stimulation (urate crystals) to produce a noxious stimulus. However, not all of the methods are selective for pain/analgesia. For example, thermal transducers produce heat, and an animal's response may be caused by temperature changes and not pain; mechanical stimulation may produce a response because of pressure of the device before activation of pain pathways; electrical stimulation can produce a response because of muscle twitching independently of pain; and chemical stimulation produces inflammation in addition to pain. Another limitation of experimental studies is that they may not extrapolate to naturally occurring pain and analgesia. A complete review of pain models is available.[9] Despite their limitations, experimental models can be helpful for providing a rational basis for use of analgesic drugs in veterinary patients. There is currently no gold standard and every model has limitations.

CLINICAL IMPRESSIONS OF ANALGESIC EFFICACY

Clinical impressions are one of the most common sources of information on drug use in veterinary medicine, especially with the advent of the Internet and discussion forums. However, clinical impressions are the least reliable sources of information on drug efficacy. Clinical impressions do not account for the placebo effect, which occurs in up to 2 in 5 animals when owners or veterinarians evaluate the animal (NADA 141-053). Clinical impressions also do not control for bias from the veterinarian or owner, both of whom think that, if they are doing something, it has to be helping the animal. Clinical impressions also do not control for naturally occurring fluctuations in the severity of pain. In addition, veterinarians may lose follow-up on a case for a variety of reasons and as such may recall treating a patient, but not know the outcome and assume a positive outcome when it may or may not have occurred.

SPECIFIC PHARMACEUTICAL THERAPIES
Polysulfated Glycosaminoglycans

Polysulfated glycosaminoglycans (PSGAGs) are an FDA-approved injectable product for the control of signs associated with noninfectious degenerative and/or traumatic arthritis of canine synovial joints. The mechanism of action of PSGAG is not known. The drug may act by decreasing catabolic enzymes within the affected joints and enhances anabolic enzymes based on in vitro studies (NADA 141-038). A placebo-controlled clinical trial in which PSGAG was administered at 4.4 mg/kg (2 mg/lb) body weight intramuscularly (IM) to dogs with traumatic or degenerative joint disease supported the approval. The PSGAG significantly improved range of motion and total orthopedic score compared with placebo at 5 weeks. The percentage of responders in the PSGAG group was significantly higher than in the placebo group (65% vs 33%) at 5 weeks.

Because PSGAG is an FDA-approved drug for dogs, it is expected to provide beneficial effects for the management of noninfectious osteoarthritis when administered at 4.4 mg/kg body weight IM twice weekly for 4 weeks. There are currently no data supporting the use of PSGAG in cats, but there are no data refuting its use in cats. There are no published safety data available in cats. The current cost of PSGAG is moderate. The results and efficacy of the approved injectable product should not, and do not, support the use of other products such as oral glucosamine formulations.

Amantadine

Amantadine is an antiviral drug, but possesses other effects, including increasing central nervous system dopamine concentrations, and it is also an N-methyl-D-aspartate (NMDA) antagonist. As an NMDA antagonist, amantadine may antagonize central pain sensitization and decrease tolerance to analgesics such as opioids. Amantadine decreased opioid consumption in postoperative human patients, reduced pain in postherpetic neuralgia in humans, and has had mixed results with neuropathic pain in humans.[10,11] Amantadine is not expected to provide analgesic effects as a sole therapy, but may enhance the analgesic effects of NSAIDs, opioids, or gabapentin/pregabalin. No FDA-approved veterinary formulations are available.

The pharmacokinetics of amantadine have been incompletely described in dogs.[12] Based on urinary excretion studies in 2 dogs, amantadine seems to be well absorbed in dogs, about 10% is metabolized to N-methylamantadine, and the half-life of amantadine was short: 5 hours after 30 mg/kg. No reports are available assessing the activity or lack thereof for the metabolite. Dogs administered amantadine 50 mg/kg every 24 hours by mouth for 30 days had negligible amounts of drug in tissue samples collected 24 hours after the last dose with the investigators concluding that a dose of amantadine is eliminated within 24 hours. In cats, the pharmacokinetics are better described, with high oral bioavailability and a short half-life: approximately 5.5 hours after 5 mg/kg by mouth.[13] In contrast, the elimination half-life in humans is 15 hours.[14] Because of the short half-life, dosing every 12 hours may need to be used in dogs and cats.

Safety studies have not specifically been reported for amantadine in dogs or cats. However, 50 mg/kg every 24 hours were administered to dogs for 30 days without lethality.

No preclinical studies of amantadine analgesic effects are available in dogs. Amantadine did not have a significant effect on oxymorphone antinociception to thermal stimulus in normal cats.[15] The lack of effect is not surprising because amantadine is expected to produce effects when pain or central sensitization is already present and is not expected to decrease acute stimulus. Therefore the lack of effect in this experimental study should not be interpreted as a lack of potential clinical effects in naturally occurring pain.

A randomized, placebo-controlled and blinded clinical trial evaluated the efficacy of adding amantadine to meloxicam for the management of NSAID-refractory hind limb osteoarthritis pain in dogs.[16] Significant improvement was noted using client-specific outcome measures for activity in the amantadine treatment group (3–5 mg/kg by mouth every 24 hours) on day 42 of treatment, but not on days 7 or 21. As mentioned previously, administration every 12 hours may be a better dosage because of the rapid elimination in dogs and may result in greater efficacy. The study evaluated amantadine in combination with only 1 NSAID so it is unclear whether the same effect would be observed with other NSAIDs. No controlled clinical trials are available for amantadine use in cats.

Based on the currently available data, amantadine (3–5 mg/kg every 24 hours) may provide benefit when added to meloxicam in dogs, but the dosing frequency of amantadine may need to be increased to every 12 hours. There are currently no data supporting the use of amantadine in cats, but there are no data refuting its use in cats. The current cost of amantadine is moderate.

Tramadol

Tramadol is FDA approved for the management of moderate to moderately severe pain in humans. Tramadol is metabolized into at least 30 different metabolites, but only tramadol, O-desmethyltramadol (ODM), and N,O-didesmethyltramadol (DDM) have been associated with pharmacologic effects.[17] Tramadol administration produces analgesia, which is partially blocked by naloxone (mu opioid antagonist), yohimbine (alpha-2 antagonist), ketanserin (serotonin 5-hydroxytryptamine [HT]-2 antagonist), and ondansetron (5HT-3 antagonist), suggesting that all 3 receptor systems contribute to the analgesic effects. Other studies have also suggested that tramadol produces antagonist effects at muscarinic M1 receptors that can be overcome by acetylcholine administration. Further studies have shown that the mu opioid effects are primarily caused by ODM with some secondary effects of DDM, whereas the serotonin and norepinephrine effects are caused by tramadol and ODM, and the antimuscarinic effects are caused by ODM.

Pharmacokinetic studies in dogs have shown that dogs do not produce ODM as a substantial metabolite after tramadol administration; however, they do produce DDM.[18] Therefore dogs are not expected to have substantial opioid effects after tramadol administration. Plasma concentrations of tramadol after administration of 10 mg/kg by mouth to dogs were slightly less than the plasma concentrations achieved in humans administered 100 mg single doses, but the concentration of ODM was 10 times less in dogs compared with humans. The elimination half-life of tramadol in dogs is more rapid (1.1 hours) compared with humans (5.6 hours). The production of DDM, which has an elimination half-life of 3.6 hours in dogs, may produce some opioid effects in dogs. Repeated doses of tramadol either decreased drug absorption or enhanced presystemic metabolism of tramadol in dogs, in which a 60% to 70% decrease in tramadol plasma concentrations resulted after just 8 days of treatment (20 mg/kg by mouth).[1] The effects of multiple-day administration on the metabolites ODM and DDM were not reported.

In contrast with dogs, cats produce high concentrations of ODM after tramadol administration and as a result have prominent opioid effects.[19] The concentrations of ODM after 5.2 mg/kg tramadol by mouth were 10 times higher than ODM concentrations in humans after 100 mg by mouth. The terminal half-life of ODM after oral tramadol in cats was 4.5 hours, suggesting that administration every 12 hours may be appropriate in cats. The plasma concentrations of tramadol and ODM were dose proportional from 0.5 to 4 mg/kg by mouth.[20] The pharmacokinetics of repeated doses of tramadol have not been reported in cats.

A pressure pain threshold model was used to assess the effects of oral tramadol (10 mg/kg by mouth) in dogs.[18] Significant increases in thresholds were observed only at 5 and 6 hours after administration. It is unclear how mechanical antinociceptive effects translate to clinical analgesic effects.

The effects of tramadol on thermal thresholds in cats have been reported.[20,21] The thermal thresholds exceeded the 95% confidence interval at 0.75, 3, and 6 hours after 1 mg/kg tramadol, but not at 1, 2, 4, 8, and 24 hours.[21] A dose titration study evaluated the effects of tramadol dosed 0.5 to 4 mg/kg by mouth in cats using a thermal threshold model. Thermal thresholds increased proportionally with increased doses.[20] The duration of increased thresholds were also related to the dose, with 2 mg/kg producing significant effects from less than 6 hours to up to 13 hours after administration, 3 mg/kg producing significant effects from 9 to 12 hours after administration, and 4 mg/kg producing significant effects from 10 to 16 hours after administration.

There are few studies assessing the effects of tramadol administration to clinical canine patients in controlled clinical trials. Only 1 study reports the effects of oral tramadol in a blinded study using positive and negative controls, and these were in patients with osteoarthritis. The incorporation of both positive and negative controls is important because an effect (perceived improvement) occurred in the placebo group using an owner-completed canine brief pain inventory questionnaire.[2] However, significant improvement was noted in the positive control group (carprofen, 2.2 mg/kg twice a day) and tramadol (4 mg/kg 3 times a day) group compared with the placebo (administered 3 times a day). Plasma concentrations of carprofen and tramadol were measured 3 hours after the first dose and last dose (14 day). The plasma concentrations of carprofen were within the expected plasma concentrations. The plasma concentrations of tramadol were low (39.3 ± 35.3 ng/mL) 3 hours after the first dose and were significantly decreased 3 hours after the last dose (7.1 ± 8.8 ng/mL), and not even detected in 4 of 11 dogs, again suggesting decreased bioavailability with multiple doses. In comparison, the plasma concentrations of tramadol in humans after 100 mg by mouth peak at 308 ng/mL 2 to 3 hours after dosing. The plasma concentrations of ODM and DDM were not reported.

There are few studies assessing the effects of tramadol administration to clinical feline patients in controlled clinical trials. Only 1 study reports the effects of tramadol using a blinded study with negative controls and these were in patients after ovariohysterectomy. Treatment groups included placebo, the NSAID vedaprofen (0.5 mg/kg by mouth), tramadol (2 mg/kg subcutaneously [SC]), and the combination of tramadol and vedaprofen.[22] Patients were evaluated with a composite pain scale. All of the patients receiving placebo and vedaprofen received rescue analgesia, 50% of the tramadol patients received rescue analgesia, and none of the vedaprofen and tramadol group received rescue analgesia. The composite pain scale was significantly lower for the combination of vedaprofen and tramadol from 1 to 56 hours after surgery, but not significantly lower in any of the other treatment groups for more than 1 time point compared with placebo.

Tramadol is overall well tolerated in dogs. Administration of single oral doses of 450 mg/kg was not fatal in an unstated number of dogs.[1] Administration of 40 mg/kg per day to 8 dogs was well tolerated for 1 year, with mydriasis and reduced body weight observed. Adverse effects of tramadol overdose include restlessness, difficulty walking, salivation, vomiting, tremors, and convulsions. Anecdotal reports suggest that diazepam is effective in controlling tramadol-induced convulsions. Similar adverse effects are expected in cats with acute tramadol overdoses.

Adverse effects such as nausea and anorexia, and occasionally sedation, can occur in dogs with routine dosages of tramadol. According to the label, tramadol may also decrease the seizure threshold in humans and as such it would be best to avoid use in animals prone to seizures. Tramadol is bitter tasting and can result in profuse salivation and retching if the animal tastes the drug. Similar adverse effects are expected in cats with routine doses of tramadol.

A case series describing 3 postoperative dogs reported higher potential of GI adverse effects when tramadol was combined with deracoxib, an NSAID, than expected from an NSAID alone.[23] There are not currently any contraindications listed for tramadol use with NSAIDs in humans. However, there is documentation of potential interactions with other drugs affecting serotonin reuptake, including selective serotonin reuptake inhibitors (eg, fluoxetine, paroxetine) and serotonin-norepinephrine reuptake inhibitors (SNRIs; eg, venlafaxine, duloxetine) increasing the risk of GI ulcers administered alone or in combination with NSAIDs.[24] In addition, a case series in humans identified that patients prone to GI adverse effects of NSAIDs had a higher risk of GI perforation caused by tramadol administered alone.[25] The mechanism of action is thought to be serotonin-enhanced gastric acid secretion through vagal stimulation. Another potential mechanism is decreased platelet aggregation caused by serotonin depletion within the platelets, because platelets do not synthesize serotonin and rely on transport to accumulate serotonin. On activation of platelets, serotonin is released, resulting in vasoconstriction and subsequent enhanced hemostasis. The risk of GI bleeding in humans administered drugs that inhibit serotonin reuptake and NSAIDs is decreased if acid-suppression therapy (eg, H2 antagonists such as famotidine or proton pump inhibitors such as omeprazole) is coadministered. Therefore it may be prudent to administer acid-suppression therapy to dogs and cats when tramadol is administered concurrently with an NSAID to decrease the risk of GI adverse effects.

The use of tramadol with other drugs that affect serotonin reuptake or metabolism should be avoided because of the risk of serotonin toxicity. Monoamine oxidase inhibitors (selegiline), tricyclic antidepressants (TCAs; eg, amitriptyline, clomipramine), selective serotonin reuptake inhibitors (fluoxetine, paroxetine), and SNRIs (venlafaxine) should not be administered concurrently with tramadol. Serotonin syndrome has been documented in dogs, with signs such as tremors, rigidity, myoclonus, seizure, hyperthermia, salivation, and even death.[26]

Because of the high concentrations of ODM in cats administered tramadol, opioid-mediated adverse effects can occur in this species. Sedation, mydriasis, dysphoria or euphoria, constipation, and vomiting can occur in cats.

There are some data supporting tramadol use in clinical veterinary patients, but more studies need to be conducted to confirm its efficacy and safety in dogs and cats. Dogs may benefit from tramadol administered 4 to 10 mg/kg by mouth 3 times a day. However, the long-term efficacy of tramadol may decrease with time. Cats may benefit from tramadol after surgery when combined with an NSAID. Other studies are needed to fully describe the potential uses of tramadol in dogs and cats.

Tramadol is not currently a Drug Enforcement Agency (DEA) scheduled drug. However, numerous US states have enacted laws requiring special handling as a potential drug of abuse, including classifying it as a schedule IV (CIV) drug. Therefore any prescribers should check with their respective boards of pharmacy to determine current requirements for tramadol prescriptions. Tramadol has a moderate potential for diversion or misuse. The current cost of tramadol is low.

Gabapentin

Gabapentin is FDA approved as an anticonvulsant and as an analgesic for postherpetic neuralgia for human use. Gabapentin enacarbil (an extended-release gabapentin ester) is also FDA approved for the treatment of restless legs syndrome in humans. Gabapentin is a structural analog of gamma-aminobutyric acid (GABA), but does not bind directly to the GABA receptors. The mechanisms for gabapentin's anticonvulsant and analgesic effects have not been definitively identified. However, gabapentin does bind to the alpha-2/delta subunit of the voltage-gated calcium channel decreasing the release of excitatory neurotransmitters. Gabapentin also increases the brain concentrations of GABA either through increased GABA synthesis, increased vesicular release, or decreased GABA metabolism. A thorough review of potential mechanisms of action of gabapentin has been published.[27]

The pharmacokinetics of gabapentin have been described in dogs[28] and cats.[29] Gabapentin exhibits less than proportional increases in plasma concentrations with increasing doses following oral administration because of saturation of active transporters in the GI tract. Gabapentin is primarily eliminated as unchanged drug in most species except dogs, in which metabolism to N-methyl-gabapentin accounts for approximately 40% of drug disposition.[30] The terminal half-life of gabapentin is short in dogs (3–4 hours) and cats (~3 hours), necessitating dosing at least every 8 hours to maintain minimum targeted concentrations associated with efficacy in humans (2 µg/mL). Therefore dosing compliance is a limitation of gabapentin therapy in dogs and cats. A dosage of 10 to 20 mg/kg every 8 hours maintains targeted concentrations in dogs and cats. The pharmacokinetics of gabapentin enacarbil have not been published in dogs or cats, therefore it is unknown whether an extended dosing interval is possible with gabapentin enacarbil in dogs or cats.

Gabapentin failed to show an analgesic effect in cats in an experimental thermal antinociceptive model at doses ranging from 5 to 30 mg/kg.[31] However, gabapentin is not expected to be efficacious in preventing acute pain, therefore the lack of effects in this experimental study do not extrapolate to lack of efficacy for clinical use in cats.

Case reports have suggested that gabapentin produced desirable effects in managing trauma and orthopedic pain in cats.[32,33] Because these were case reports, positive and negative controls were not included. Case studies have been published in dogs suggesting efficacy as an anticonvulsant when combined with phenobarbital and bromide.[34,35]

No controlled clinical trials have been published evaluating the efficacy of gabapentin as an analgesic or anticonvulsant in dogs or cats, therefore the evidence for its use is low. However, some reports of postoperative use in dogs suggested it was not effective.[36,37] Because inappropriate dosages (5–10 mg/kg every 12 hours) were used, meaningful conclusions could not be drawn from these studies.

Adverse effects of gabapentin can include sedation and ataxia and are more likely when administered at higher dosages or when combined with other drugs that produce similar adverse effects. Abrupt discontinuation after chronic administration of gabapentin may result in withdrawal and seizures. It is suggested to taper the dose over the course of 1 week when discontinuation of chronic administration is needed. Although the oral liquid formulation contains xylitol, which can be toxic to dogs, the concentration in the solution is low enough that routine dosing of gabapentin is unlikely to result in xylitol toxicity. However, administering multiple products containing xylitol may increase the potential for xylitol toxicity.

The overall evidence for gabapentin use as an analgesic in dogs and cats is low. Pharmacokinetic studies suggest dosages of 10 to 20 mg/kg every 8 hours for dogs and cats. However, there are no controlled clinical trials using appropriate doses supporting or refuting the use of gabapentin as an analgesic. The current cost of gabapentin is low.

Pregabalin

Pregabalin is an FDA-approved anticonvulsant and an analgesic for diabetic neuropathy, postherpetic, and fibromyalgia pain in humans. Extralabel use of pregabalin in humans has suggested that it also decreases opiate consumption after surgery and decreases postoperative nausea and vomiting.[38] There are no published studies assessing pregabalin for osteoarthritis pain. There are no veterinary-approved pregabalin formulations. The mechanism by which pregabalin produces anticonvulsant and analgesic effects has not been definitively identified. However, pregabalin does bind to the alpha-2/delta subunit of the voltage-gated calcium channel (similar to gabapentin), decreasing the release of several neurotransmitters including glutamate and substance P.

The pharmacokinetics of pregabalin have been described in the dog,[39] but not in the cat. In most species, pregabalin is eliminated intact in the urine, but approximately 45% of the administered dose is metabolized to N-methyl-pregabalin in the dog. Pregabalin seems to be well absorbed after oral administration to dogs, with a terminal half-life of approximately 7 hours, suggesting that a dosing schedule of every 12 hours may be appropriate, which is an advantage compared with gabapentin.

Sedation and ataxia are potential adverse effects. Abrupt discontinuation in humans can result in withdrawal and seizures. It is suggested to taper the dose over the course of 1 week when discontinuation after chronic administration is required. Visual disturbances including blurred vision have been reported in humans. Peripheral edema unrelated to changes in blood pressure is a reported adverse effect in humans. Life-threatening angioedema has also been reported in humans.

Pharmacokinetic studies suggest a dosage of 4 mg/kg by mouth every 12 hours in dogs. No case reports, experimental data, or clinical efficacy data are available in dogs or cats. Therefore the evidence for its use is low in dogs and cats. Pregabalin is a DEA CV drug and has a low to moderate potential for diversion or misuse. The current cost of pregabalin is high.

Codeine

Codeine is an FDA-approved mu opioid agonist for the relief of mild to moderately severe pain in humans. Codeine tablets are available as a sole ingredient or in combination with other drugs, including acetaminophen. Codeine is well absorbed in humans (60% oral bioavailability) and is metabolized to numerous metabolites, with codeine-6-glucuronide, norcodeine, and morphine contributing to opioid effects.[40,41]

In contrast with humans, the oral bioavailability of codeine in dogs is 4% and morphine was not detected in measurable concentrations.[3] However, codeine-6-glucuronide, which is an active opioid metabolite, was formed in high concentrations and may provide analgesic effects in dogs.[41]

The urinary elimination of codeine was evaluated in cats after administration of 20 mg/kg SC codeine.[42] Norcodeine was identified as the major metabolite in cats, but neither the plasma concentrations nor the elimination half-lives of codeine and norcodeine were reported for cats. Further pharmacokinetic studies of codeine are warranted in cats.

Experimental models using electrical stimulation of tooth pulp in dogs showed that the antinociceptive effect of 2 mg/kg SC codeine was similar to 0.1 mg/kg morphine SC, suggesting that parenteral codeine was a low-potency analgesic with a short duration (2 hours) in dogs.[43] Oral codeine (20 mg/kg) produced depression of hind limb reflexes in dogs with chronic spinal disorders that was similar to morphine 0.5 mg/kg, but it is unclear how the study applies clinically to painful dogs.[44]

Regardless, the analgesic/antinociceptive effects of codeine were low with regard to efficacy and potency compared with parenteral morphine.

There are no reports of oral codeine efficacy in clinical cases or controlled clinical studies. There are no reports of the antinociceptive/analgesic effects of codeine in cats in experimental studies or clinical cases. Therefore the evidence for use of oral codeine in dogs and cats is low. Although codeine dosages have been recommended at 1.1 to 2.2 mg/kg by mouth every 6 to 12 hours, data are lacking to support those recommendations. It is important to remember that codeine formulations with acetaminophen can be safely administered to dogs, but result in acetaminophen toxicity in cats. Therefore only codeine formulations that do not contain acetaminophen should be used in cats. Codeine as a sole ingredient is a DEA CII drug and combinations of codeine with acetaminophen are CIII drugs. Codeine formulations have a high potential for diversion or misuse. The current cost of oral codeine formulations is low.

Hydrocodone

Hydrocodone is a mu opioid agonist that is FDA approved as an antitussive and analgesic in humans. Hydrocodone is only available as combination products, which is likely to curb its potential for abuse. The drug combinations that can be administered to dogs include hydrocodone with homatropine and hydrocodone with acetaminophen. The drug combination that can be administered to cats is hydrocodone with homatropine.

Hydrocodone pharmacokinetics have been reported in dogs dosed with the commercially available hydrocodone/acetaminophen tablets.[3] Oral administration of hydrocodone, 0.5 mg/kg by mouth, resulted in plasma concentrations of hydrocodone and hydromorphone (a hydrocodone metabolite) that persisted for at least 8 hours at concentrations greater than those considered therapeutic in humans. Tablets can be quartered with reasonable accuracy within 22% of the expected hydrocodone content, whereas half-tablet fractions were within 10% of the expected content.[3]

There have been no reported experimental studies or clinical trials evaluating the efficacy of oral hydrocodone in dogs or cats. Hydrocodone is currently a DEA CIII drug and has a high potential for diversion or misuse. The current cost of hydrocodone combinations is low.

TCAs

TCAs such as amitriptyline are considered first-line therapeutics for neuropathic pain in humans. Their efficacy has been shown primarily in patients with postherpetic neuralgia.[45] Additional studies have indicated likely efficacy in central neuropathic pain conditions such as poststroke pain, but not spinal cord injury. TCAs were not superior to placebo for rheumatoid arthritis, but were superior to placebo for ankylosing spondylitis and chronic low back pain.

TCAs produce analgesia through multiple mechanisms. They produce serotonin and norepinephrine reuptake inhibition, NMDA antagonism, and voltage-gated sodium channel blockade; they enhance the activity of adenosine and $GABA_B$ receptors; and they have antiinflammatory effects.[45] Amitriptyline is the TCA most consistently reported to produce analgesic effects in human neuropathic pain.

Adverse effects of TCAs are primarily caused by their effects as muscarinic antagonists, antihistamines, and alpha-1 antagonists. As such, adverse effects such as xerostomia, polyuria, polydipsia, urine retention, blurred vision (antimuscarinic), sedation (antihistamine), hypotension (alpha-1 antagonism) can occur with TCAs. In humans, weight gain, seizures, agitation, and cardiac arrhythmias can occur. TCAs have not been associated with GI ulceration. In contrast with SNRIs, TCAs have not been reported to affect platelet function. TCAs have been associated with bone marrow suppression including agranulocytosis, leukopenia, and thrombocytopenia.

The pharmacokinetics of oral amitriptyline were recently reported in dogs.[46] The pharmacokinetics after a dose of 3 to 4 mg/kg resulted in a peak concentration of 126 ng/mL at 2 hours and a short half-life of 5 hours. The active metabolite, nortriptyline, was not assessed. The optimum concentrations of amitriptyline plus nortriptyline in humans are 60 to 220 ng/mL, suggesting that the dose of 3 to 4 mg/kg administered every 12 hours may produce targeted concentrations but, again, without studies assessing nortriptyline concentrations in dogs it is difficult to make dosage recommendations. However, these data may indicate that higher doses of amitriptyline may be needed in dogs than are currently recommended (1–2 mg/kg every 12 hours).

Partial pharmacokinetics of oral amitriptyline in cats are reported after 5 mg per cat (1.3–1.4 mg/kg) using a nonspecific immunoassay that measured amitriptyline and any metabolites (active or inactive).[47] A mean maximum plasma concentration (CMAX) of 61 ng/mL was achieved at 2 hours, and that decreased to about 20 ng/mL at 12 hours. Plasma concentrations of a pluronic lecithin organogel formulation of amitriptyline resulted in low and undetectable concentrations, suggesting it was not a reasonable route of administration.

There are no experimental studies are clinical trials assessing the efficacy of TCAs for canine pain. A case series reported the effects of amitriptyline in 3 dogs with suspected neuropathic pain in which 2 of three were reported to be improved. There are no studies or case reports assessing the efficacy of TCAs in feline pain. The currently recommended doses of amitriptyline, 1 to 2.2 mg/kg every 12 hours, may be too low. The current cost of amitriptyline is low.

SNRIs

SNRIs such as venlafaxine and duloxetine have analgesic effects in neuropathic and osteoarthritis pain in humans.[45,48] Duloxetine is FDA approved to treat humans with chronic low back pain and chronic osteoarthritis, but may take several weeks to achieve the desired effect.

The pharmacokinetics of venlafaxine have been reported in dogs.[49] Oral administration of 4 mg/kg results in a CMAX of 480 ng/mL at 2 hours after administration, with a terminal half-life of 3 hours. The short half-life suggests at least twice-daily, and maybe every 8 hours, administration is needed. The oral bioavailability is about 50%. The active metabolite, desvenlafaxine is apparently not produced in dogs, therefore, in contrast with humans, pharmacologic effects are only caused by the parent drug, venlafaxine. The pharmacokinetics of venlafaxine have not been reported in cats.

Some pharmacokinetic parameters of duloxetine in dogs have been reported as part of the human drug approval by the European Medicines Agency. The oral bioavailability of duloxetine is only 5% in dogs and the terminal half-life is about 4 hours. Although dose-proportional pharmacokinetics are reported up to 30 mg/kg, the plasma concentrations or CMAX were not reported. During toxicology studies, vomiting was dose related and the dose-limiting effect, but other adverse effects such as anorexia, abnormal stools, and mydriasis were reported. Hepatic changes occurred in dogs treated with 30 mg/kg, including microsomal induction (which may further shorten the half-life) and increased liver weight. The unfavorable pharmacokinetic profile of duloxetine favors venlafaxine for further assessment in dogs at this time. The pharmacokinetics of duloxetine have not been reported in cats.

There are no studies reporting the pharmacodynamics effects of venlafaxine or duloxetine in dogs or cats using experimental models, clinical cases, or controlled clinical trials. The cost of the SNRIs are currently much greater than the cost of amitriptyline.

Glucosamine and Chondroitin

Glucosamine and chondroitin are nutritional supplements that are anecdotally recommended for use in patients with osteoarthritis. The purported mechanism of action is to support cartilage matrix production and minimize cartilage degradation. There are currently no FDA-approved formulations of glucosamine or chondroitin for dogs or cats.

There has been only 1 published clinical trial incorporating both positive and negative controls that evaluated the efficacy of glucosamine and chondroitin supplements in dogs. Compared with placebo, no significant effects could be attributed to glucosamine and chondroitin, but significant improvements were shown for both carprofen and meloxicam.[50]

Current literature does not support the use of glucosamine and chondroitin supplements for the control of osteoarthritis pain in dogs.

Morphine, Oxycodone, Methadone

The pharmacokinetics of oral morphine,[51] oxycodone,[52] and methadone,[53] have been reported in dogs. The pharmacokinetics indicate low oral bioavailability and plasma concentrations and short half-lives, suggesting that these opioids do not produce a consistent clinical effect in dogs. Because of the low, variable, and inconsistent absorption of these drugs administered orally in dogs, simple increases in dose are unlikely to produce consistent opioid effects. No studies have reported analgesic effects of oral morphine, oxycodone, or methadone in dogs in either experimental studies or clinical studies.

The pharmacokinetics or analgesic effects of oral morphine, oxycodone, or methadone have not been reported in cats. Because the pharmacokinetics of intravenous administration in cats are similar to those reported in dogs, it is likely these drugs have a low oral bioavailability and lack of consistent clinical effects in cats as well.

Morphine, methadone, and oxycodone are DEA CII drugs and have high potentials for diversion and misuse. The amount of evidence available for these drugs administered orally does not support their use in dogs and cats.

REFERENCES

1. Matthiesen T, Wöhrmann T, Coogan TP, et al. The experimental toxicology of tramadol: an overview. Toxicol Lett 1998;95:63–71.
2. Malek S, Sample SJ, Schwartz Z, et al. Effect of analgesic therapy on clinical outcome measures in a randomized controlled trial using client-owned dogs with hip osteoarthritis. BMC Vet Res 2012;8:185.
3. KuKanich B, Spade J. Pharmacokinetics of hydrocodone and hydromorphone after oral hydrocodone in healthy greyhound dogs. Vet J 2012. http://dx.doi.org/10.1016/j.tvjl.2012.09.008. pii:S1090–0233(12)00393-0.
4. KuKanich B. Pharmacokinetics of acetaminophen, codeine, and the codeine metabolites morphine and codeine-6-glucuronide in healthy greyhound dogs. J Vet Pharmacol Ther 2010;33:15–21.
5. Papich MG, Alcorn J. Absorption of diazepam after its rectal administration in dogs. Am J Vet Res 1995;56:1629–36.

6. Neirinckx E, Vervaet C, De Boever S, et al. Species comparison of oral bioavailability, first-pass metabolism and pharmacokinetics of acetaminophen. Res Vet Sci 2010;89:113–9.
7. Ritschel WA, Neub M, Denson DD. Meperidine pharmacokinetics following intravenous, peroral and buccal administration in beagle dogs. Methods Find Exp Clin Pharmacol 1987;9:811–5.
8. Shott S. Designing studies that answer questions. J Am Vet Med Assoc 2011; 238:55–8.
9. Le Bars D, Gozariu M, Cadden SW. Animal models of nociception. Pharmacol Rev 2001;53:597–652.
10. Fisher K, Coderre TJ, Hagen NA. Targeting the N-methyl-D-aspartate receptor for chronic pain management. Preclinical animal studies, recent clinical experience and future research directions. J Pain Symptom Manage 2000;20:358–73.
11. Bujak-Giżycka B, Kącka K, Suski M, et al. Beneficial effect of amantadine on postoperative pain reduction and consumption of morphine in patients subjected to elective spine surgery. Pain Med 2012;13:459–65.
12. Bleidner WE, Harmon JB, Hewes WE, et al. Absorption, distribution and excretion of amantadine hydrochloride. J Pharmacol Exp Ther 1965;150:484–90.
13. Siao KT, Pypendop BH, Stanley SD, et al. Pharmacokinetics of amantadine in cats. J Vet Pharmacol Ther 2011;34:599–604.
14. Aoki FY, Sitar DS. Effects of chronic amantadine hydrochloride ingestion on its and acetaminophen pharmacokinetics in young adults. J Clin Pharmacol 1992;32:24–7.
15. Siao KT, Pypendop BH, Escobar A, et al. Effect of amantadine on oxymorphone-induced thermal antinociception in cats. J Vet Pharmacol Ther 2012;35:169–74.
16. Lascelles BD, Gaynor JS, Smith ES, et al. Amantadine in a multimodal analgesic regimen for alleviation of refractory osteoarthritis pain in dogs. J Vet Intern Med 2008;22:53–9.
17. Grond S, Sablotzki A. Clinical pharmacology of tramadol. Clin Pharmacokinet 2004;43:879–923.
18. KuKanich B, Papich MG. Pharmacokinetics and antinociceptive effects of oral tramadol hydrochloride administration in greyhounds. Am J Vet Res 2011;72: 256–62.
19. Pypendop BH, Ilkiw JE. Pharmacokinetics of tramadol, and its metabolite O-desmethyl-tramadol, in cats. J Vet Pharmacol Ther 2008;31:52–9.
20. Pypendop BH, Siao KT, Ilkiw JE. Effects of tramadol hydrochloride on the thermal threshold in cats. Am J Vet Res 2009;70:1465–70.
21. Steagall PV, Taylor PM, Brondani JT, et al. Antinociceptive effects of tramadol and acepromazine in cats. J Feline Med Surg 2008;10:24–31.
22. Brondani JT, Loureiro Luna SP, Beier SL, et al. Analgesic efficacy of perioperative use of vedaprofen, tramadol or their combination in cats undergoing ovariohysterectomy. J Feline Med Surg 2009;11:420–9.
23. Case JB, Fick JL, Rooney MB. Proximal duodenal perforation in three dogs following deracoxib administration. J Am Anim Hosp Assoc 2010;46:255–8.
24. Andrade C, Sandarsh S, Chethan KB, et al. Serotonin reuptake inhibitor antidepressants and abnormal bleeding: a review for clinicians and a reconsideration of mechanisms. J Clin Psychiatry 2010;71:1565–75.
25. Tørring ML, Riis A, Christensen S, et al. Perforated peptic ulcer and short-term mortality among tramadol users. Br J Clin Pharmacol 2008;65:565–72.
26. Mohammad-Zadeh LF, Moses L, Gwaltney-Brant SM. Serotonin: a review. J Vet Pharmacol Ther 2008;31:187–99.

27. Sills GJ. The mechanisms of action of gabapentin and pregabalin. Curr Opin Pharmacol 2006;6:108–13.
28. KuKanich B, Cohen RL. Pharmacokinetics of oral gabapentin in greyhound dogs. Vet J 2011;187:133–5.
29. Siao KT, Pypendop BH, Ilkiw JE. Pharmacokinetics of gabapentin in cats. Am J Vet Res 2010;71:817–21.
30. Vollmer KO, von Hodenberg A, Kölle EU. Pharmacokinetics and metabolism of gabapentin in rat, dog and man. Arzneimittelforschung 1986;36:830–9.
31. Pypendop BH, Siao KT, Ilkiw JE. Thermal antinociceptive effect of orally administered gabapentin in healthy cats. Am J Vet Res 2010;71:1027–32.
32. Lorenz ND, Comerford EJ, Iff I. Long-term use of gabapentin for musculoskeletal disease and trauma in three cats. J Feline Med Surg 2013;15:507–12.
33. Vettorato E, Corletto F. Gabapentin as part of multi-modal analgesia in two cats suffering multiple injuries. Vet Anaesth Analg 2011;38:518–20.
34. Platt SR, Adams V, Garosi LS, et al. Treatment with gabapentin of 11 dogs with refractory idiopathic epilepsy. Vet Rec 2006;159:881–4.
35. Govendir M, Perkins M, Malik R. Improving seizure control in dogs with refractory epilepsy using gabapentin as an adjunctive agent. Aust Vet J 2005;83: 602–8.
36. Aghighi SA, Tipold A, Piechotta M, et al. Assessment of the effects of adjunctive gabapentin on postoperative pain after intervertebral disc surgery in dogs. Vet Anaesth Analg 2012;39:636–46.
37. Wagner AE, Mich PM, Uhrig SR, et al. Clinical evaluation of perioperative administration of gabapentin as an adjunct for postoperative analgesia in dogs undergoing amputation of a forelimb. J Am Vet Med Assoc 2010;236:751–6.
38. Zhang J, Ho KY, Wang Y. Efficacy of pregabalin in acute postoperative pain: a meta-analysis. Br J Anaesth 2011;106:454–62.
39. Salazar V, Dewey CW, Schwark W, et al. Pharmacokinetics of single-dose oral pregabalin administration in normal dogs. Vet Anaesth Analg 2009;36:574–80.
40. Fraser HF, Isbell H, Vanhorn GD. Human pharmacology and addiction liability of norcodeine. J Pharmacol Exp Ther 1960;129:172–7.
41. Lötsch J, Skarke C, Schmidt H, et al. Evidence for morphine-independent central nervous opioid effects after administration of codeine: contribution of other codeine metabolites. Clin Pharmacol Ther 2006;79:35–48.
42. Yeh SY, Woods LA. Excretion of codeine and its metabolites by dogs, rabbits and cats. Arch Int Pharmacodyn Ther 1971;191:231–42.
43. Skingle M, Tyers MB. Further studies on opiate receptors that mediate antinociception: tooth pulp stimulation in the dog. Br J Pharmacol 1980;70:323–7.
44. Martin WR, Eades CG, Fraser HF, et al. Use of hindlimb reflexes of the chronic spinal dog for comparing analgesics. J Pharmacol Exp Ther 1964;144:8–11.
45. Dharmshaktu P, Tayal V, Kalra BS. Efficacy of antidepressants as analgesics: a review. J Clin Pharmacol 2012;52:6–17.
46. Kukes VG, Kondratenko SN, Savelyeva MI, et al. Experimental and clinical pharmacokinetics of amitryptiline: comparative analysis. Bull Exp Biol Med 2009; 147:434–7.
47. Mealey KL, Peck KE, Bennett BS, et al. Systemic absorption of amitriptyline and buspirone after oral and transdermal administration to healthy cats. J Vet Intern Med 2004;18:43–6.
48. Sullivan M, Bentley S, Fan MY, et al. A single-blind placebo run-in study of venlafaxine XR for activity-limiting osteoarthritis pain. Pain Med 2009;10:806–12.

49. Howell SR, Hicks DR, Scatina JA, et al. Pharmacokinetics of venlafaxine and O-desmethylvenlafaxine in laboratory animals. Xenobiotica 1994;24:315–27.
50. Moreau M, Dupuis J, Bonneau NH, et al. Clinical evaluation of a nutraceutical, carprofen and meloxicam for the treatment of dogs with osteoarthritis. Vet Rec 2003;152:323–9.
51. KuKanich B, Lascelles BD, Papich MG. Pharmacokinetics of morphine and plasma concentrations of morphine-6-glucuronide following morphine administration to dogs. J Vet Pharmacol Ther 2005;28:371–6.
52. Weinstein SH, Gaylord JC. Determination of oxycodone in plasma and identification of a major metabolite. J Pharm Sci 1979;68:527–8.
53. KuKanich B, Lascelles BD, Aman AM, et al. The effects of inhibiting cytochrome P450 3A, p-glycoprotein, and gastric acid secretion on the oral bioavailability of methadone in dogs. J Vet Pharmacol Ther 2005;28:461–6.

Update
Seizure Management in Small Animal Practice

Karen R. Muñana, DVM, MS

KEYWORDS

- Epilepsy • Antiepileptic drug • Pharmacology • Dog • Cat

KEY POINTS

- Seizures are the most common neurologic condition encountered in small animal practice and arise from an imbalance of excitatory and inhibitory mechanisms in the brain.
- Epilepsy refers to recurrent seizures of any cause. Successful management of epilepsy requires knowledge of the pharmacologic properties of available antiepileptic medications, regular patient evaluations to assess response to therapy and monitor for adverse effects, and thorough client education to ensure that goals and expectations of therapy are understood.
- Conventional antiepileptic medications used in dogs and cats include phenobarbital and bromide. These drugs are efficacious but have a narrow therapeutic range such that side effects are common.
- Novel antiepileptic drugs used in dogs and cats include gabapentin, zonisamide, levetiracetam, and pregabalin. These drugs tend to have a wide therapeutic range, but little is currently known about their efficacy in dogs and cats.
- The successful management of an epileptic dog should include recommendations for emergency care of seizures at home. This typically consists of administration of a benzodiazepine if prolonged or repetitive seizures occur and can also include pulse therapy with an oral antiepileptic drug.

Seizures are the most common neurologic condition encountered in small animal practice, with an estimated prevalence in a referral hospital population of 1% to 2% in dogs[1,2] and 0.5% to 3.5% in cats.[1-3] Seizures are transient paroxysmal disturbances in brain function that result from an imbalance between excitatory and inhibitory neurotransmission in the brain. The resulting neuronal excitation can be identified by characteristic epileptiform activity on electroencephalography and is typically accompanied by clinical manifestations. These clinical manifestations can be expressed as alterations of consciousness, behavioral changes, involuntary motor activity, and autonomic discharge, resulting in salivation, urination, and defecation.

Department of Clinical Sciences, College of Veterinary Medicine, North Carolina State University, 1060 William Moore Drive, Raleigh, NC 27607, USA
E-mail address: karen_munana@ncsu.edu

Vet Clin Small Anim 43 (2013) 1127–1147
http://dx.doi.org/10.1016/j.cvsm.2013.04.008
vetsmall.theclinics.com

PATHOPHYSIOLOGY

Seizure activity is characterized at the neuronal level by 2 primary features, hyper-excitability and hypersynchrony. A hyperexcitable state can result from 4 general mechanisms[4]: (1) derangements of cellular metabolism that lead to excessive depo-larization of the neuronal membrane (eg, failure of the Na+/K+-ATPase pump or changes in voltage gated ion channels); (2) decrease in inhibitory neurotransmission, such as that mediated by γ-aminobutyric acid (GABA); (3) increase in excitatory neuro-transmission, such as that mediated by glutamate; and (4) alteration of local ion concentrations that favor membrane depolarization. Electrical fields created by neuronal activation can increase the excitability of neighboring neurons via non-synaptic (ephaptic) interactions and through the activation of recurrent excitatory collateral fibers, contributing to a hypersynchronous state.

EPILEPSY CLASSIFICATION

Epilepsy is a general term that refers to a clinical disorder characterized by recurrent seizures of any cause. In order to better characterize this diverse group of disorders, epilepsy is further classified with respect to cause. The International League Against Epilepsy has recently revised its classification scheme for human epilepsy (**Table 1**).[5] Universally accepted epilepsy terminology does not exist in veterinary medicine, although the classification scheme has generally followed International League Against Epilepsy guidelines. The terms, *idiopathic epilepsy, reactive epilepsy, symptomatic epilepsy,* and *probable symptomatic epilepsy,* are most commonly used (see **Table 1**). Idiopathic epilepsy typically has an age on onset in dogs of 1 to 5 years, although dogs outside of this age range have been described. There is evidence to support a heritable basis for disease in the Australian shepherd,[6] beagle,[7] Belgian Tervuren,[8] Bernese mountain dog,[9] border collie,[10] dachshund,[11] dalmatian,[12] English springer spaniel,[13] German shepherd,[14] golden retriever,[15] Irish wolfhound,[16] kees-hond,[17] Labrador retriever,[18] lagotto Romagnolo,[19] Shetland sheepdog,[20] standard poodle,[21] and vizsla.[22]

Table 1
Epilepsy classification schemes commonly used in human and veterinary medicine

Human Epilepsy Classification	Definition	Analogous Veterinary Classification
Genetic epilepsy	Chronic recurring seizures for which there is no underlying cause other than a presumed genetic predisposition	Idiopathic epilepsy
Metabolic epilepsy	Distinct metabolic condition or disease demonstrated to be associated with an increased risk of developing seizures	Reactive epilepsy
Structural epilepsy	Congenital or acquired structural lesion in the brain associated with an increased risk of developing seizures	Symptomatic epilepsy
Epilepsy of unknown cause	Nature of underlying cause is as yet unknown	Probable symptomatic epilepsy Cryptogenic epilepsy

GENERAL PRINCIPLES OF THERAPY
Initiating Treatment

Dogs with symptomatic epilepsy should have treatment directed at the underlying cause, if possible. This is particularly important if a metabolic cause is identified, because reactive seizures are often refractory to antiepileptic drug treatment if the primary cause is not addressed.

Common guidelines exist as to when to initiate antiepileptic drug therapy. Clinicians must also take into consideration, however, the general health of the patient as well as the owner's lifestyle, financial limitations, and comfort with the proposed therapeutic regimen. A final decision should be made on a case-by-case basis with these factors in mind. As a general rule, the author recommends initiation of treatment when any of the following criteria is present:

- Seizure frequency is ≥ 1 a month.
- There is a history of cluster seizures or status epilepticus.
- The seizure itself or the postictal signs are considered especially severe.
- The owner has a strong desire to treat the seizures regardless of the frequency or severity.

Therapeutic recommendations have been based on the belief that long-term seizure management is most successful when antiepileptic therapy is initiated early in the course of disease. An epidemiologic study of Labrador retrievers with epilepsy demonstrated that dogs with a low total number of seizures prior to treatment responded better to antiepileptic therapy than dogs that had multiple seizures before treatment was initiated.[23] Similarly, among humans with epilepsy, patients with the greatest number of seizures prior to initiation of treatment are more likely to respond poorly to antiepileptic therapy.[24] Historically, this phenomenon has been attributed to kindling, in which seizure activity leads to intensification of subsequent seizures. There is little clinical evidence, however, to substantiate that kindling plays a role in either dogs[25] or humans[26] with recurrent seizures. Rather, recent epidemiologic data suggest that there are differences in the inherent severity of epilepsy among individuals, and these differences influence a patient's response to medication and long-term outcome.[27] Breed-related differences in epilepsy severity have been described in dogs, with a moderate to severe clinical course reported in Australian shepherds[6] and border collies,[10] whereas a less severe form of disease has been described in collies.[28]

Client Education

Client education is key to the successful management of epilepsy. Pet owners should have a thorough understanding of the goals and expectations of treatment prior to initiating therapy. Key points that should be discussed with owners are outlined:

- Many animals do not become seizure-free with treatment. Rather, a realistic goal might be control of seizures to an acceptable level that allows for the best quality of life.
- Antiepileptic drug therapy is lifelong in most instances.
- Managing a pet with epilepsy requires a time commitment. A lifestyle adjustment might be needed to assure that a pet receives medication at the prescribed interval each day, because even 1 missed dosage of medication can precipitate seizures in some individuals.
- There is a considerable financial commitment involved in managing a pet with epilepsy. In addition to the cost of medication, pets should have a physical

examination and laboratory evaluation performed at minimum on an annual basis.

- Antiepileptic drugs are not without side effects, and a reduction of seizures must be balanced with minimizing drug-related adverse effects.
- Owners must be committed to the treatment at the onset of therapy. Otherwise, client compliance might become a problem and treatment is less likely to be successful.

Choosing an Antiepileptic Drug

Factors to consider when choosing an antiepileptic medication include

- Mechanism of action
- Efficacy
- Adverse effects of the medication
- Potential for drug interactions
- Frequency of administration (which might influence compliance)
- Cost

Regardless of the drug used, optimal treatment results are best achieved by adopting a systematic approach to seizure management (**Fig. 1**). In general, administration of a single antiepileptic drug rather than a combination of drugs is preferred at the onset of treatment, because this avoids drug-drug interactions and provides a simpler regimen that may improve compliance.[29] Adequate treatment response is assessed based on seizure frequency once the drug has reached steady-state concentrations, serum drug concentrations when applicable, and the severity of side effects. If seizures remain inadequately controlled in an animal with serum drug concentrations within the low therapeutic range and no evidence of medication-related side effects, the dosage of the drug should be increased. A drug should not be considered to have failed until maximum dosage or therapeutic serum concentrations have been attained, or unacceptable side effects occur. If the single agent does not adequately control seizures at optimal dosages, then a second drug should be added and attempts made to gradually wean the first drug. If this is unsuccessful, polytherapy should be maintained. When choosing an add-on drug, it is preferred to use drugs with differing mechanisms of action that can be administered concurrently without the potential for drug interactions.

Assessing Safety and Efficacy

A fundamental tenet of evidence-based medicine is that the practice of medicine should be based on valid, clinically relevant research data. Guidelines for use of antiepileptic drugs in human medicine are routinely based on randomized controlled studies. In contrast, most of the data available on efficacy and safety of antiepileptic therapy in veterinary medicine are derived from retrospective or open-label studies. An analysis of 3 randomized controlled trials involving dogs with canine epilepsy demonstrated that 30% of dogs experienced a 50% or greater reduction in seizures with placebo administration.[30] Retrospective studies and open-label trials cannot account for a placebo effect and, consequently, it is likely that the efficacy data from such studies are overstated.

Monitoring Response to Therapy

Epilepsy is a chronic disease, and clinicians should view its management as such. Ideally, the goal of therapy is seizure remission; however, this cannot be achieved in most instances. Less than half of all epileptic dogs are able to maintain a seizure-free status without experiencing adverse effects from the medication.[31]

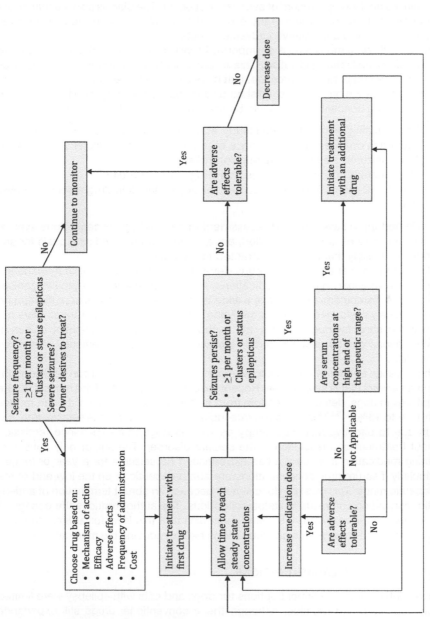

Fig. 1. Algorithm outlining the approach to the use of antiepileptic drugs in dogs and cats.

Consequently, the primary aim of treatment is to optimize control of seizures while minimizing the adverse effects of the antiepileptic medication.

Epilepsy management depends to a large extent on accurate owner observation, particularly when assessing the efficacy of therapy. Owners should be instructed to maintain a diary to keep a record of seizures that occur. The diary is also a useful place for the owner to record whether any doses of medication are not administered as scheduled and note any observed adverse effects.

Therapeutic drug monitoring is an important tool in evaluating both the efficacy and toxicity of antiepileptic medication. This is particularly important in drugs, such as phenobarbital and potassium bromide, that have a narrow therapeutic index, for which a therapeutic range has been established and levels are routinely monitored. In such instances, drug concentrations should be measured at the following times:

- After initiating treatment, once steady-state concentrations are achieved
- After each dosage adjustment, once steady-state concentrations are achieved
- When seizured are not adequately controlled
- When there is concern about possible drug-related toxicity
- At 6- to 12-month intervals to screen for any changes in drug disposition over time

It is important to have a regular assessment of serum drug concentrations even at times when seizures are well controlled, because this can be used as a basis for any changes in therapy that might be warranted in the future.

Many of the newer antiepileptic drugs developed for the treatment of humans are now used in veterinary patients. Medications, such as gabapentin, pregabalin, zonisamide, and levetiracetam, tend to have a wide therapeutic index, and serum monitoring is not routinely performed in human medicine. Although therapeutic ranges have not been established for dogs or cats, the author thinks that measurement of serum concentrations can be useful in certain instances to assess the efficacy of a given medication.

The question frequently arises as to when antiepileptic medication can be discontinued in an animal that is seizure-free. Recent research suggests that the remission rate of epilepsy in dogs, defined as freedom from seizures for a minimum of 1 year, ranges from 15% to 18%.[10,32] This remission rate includes dogs in which the seizure-free status is due to effective medical therapy as well as dogs that experience remission without treatment or a resolution of the seizure disorder. The author only considers weaning medication if an animal has experienced no seizures for a year or longer, particularly if serum drug concentrations are subtherapeutic or on the low end of the therapeutic range. This must be done slowly because an abrupt termination of antiepileptic medication can result in status epilepticus. The author reduces the dosage of medication by approximately 25% and maintains it at this level for at least the time required to reach steady-state concentrations before reducing the medication further.

PHARMACOLOGIC TREATMENT OPTIONS

Until recently, primary treatment options for dogs and cats with epilepsy were limited to phenobarbital and bromide. Although these conventional drugs still experience widespread use in veterinary practice, several new antiepileptic drugs have been developed for use in humans over the past 20 years that are now used in the treatment of canine and feline epilepsy. By providing additional treatment options, the availability of these novel drugs has made a tremendous impact on the management of epilepsy in dogs and cats. The optimum use of these drugs has yet to be established in veterinary patients. Although their relative efficacy has not been determined, they tend to have a wide therapeutic index and offer the potential of minimizing adverse effects of treatment. Properties of the antiepileptic drugs used to treat dogs and cats are summarized in **Tables 2** and **3**.

Phenobarbital

Mechanism of action

The primary mechanism by which phenobarbital exerts it antiepileptic effect is potentiation of inhibition at the postsynaptic level through action on the $GABA_A$ receptor. Specifically, phenobarbital enhances receptor-mediated chloride currents by prolonging the opening of postsynaptic chloride channels, resulting in increased intracellular chloride concentration and subsequent hyperpolarization of the cell membrane.[33] At higher concentrations, phenobarbital also causes a presynaptic reduction of calcium dependent action potentials, which might also contribute to its antiepileptic effect.[34]

Table 2
Summary of pharmacologic properties of antiepileptic drugs used as maintenance therapy in dogs

Drug	Recommended Starting Oral Dose	Time to Steady-State Concentration (Days)	Route of Elimination	Reported Adverse Effects
Phenobarbital	2.5–3.0 mg/kg q 12 h	10–14	Hepatic metabolism—CYP enzyme system	Sedation, ataxia Polyphagia Polyuria/ polydipsia Hepatotoxicity Bone marrow suppression Hyperexcitability
Bromide	30 mg/kg q 24 h	100–200	Renal excretion	Sedation, ataxia Vomiting Polyuria/ polydipsia Polyphagia Pancreatitis
Gabapentin	10–20 mg/kg q 6–8 h	1	Renal excretion; portion undergoes hepatic metabolism	Sedation, ataxia
Zonisamide	5–10 mg/kg q 12 h	3–4	Hepatic metabolism—CYP enzyme system	Sedation, ataxia Loss of appetite
Levetiracetam	20 mg/kg q 8 h	1	Primarily renal excretion; some enzymatic hydrolysis	Sedation, ataxia
Pregabalin	3–4 mg/kg q 8 h	1–2	Renal excretion; portion undergoes hepatic metabolism	Sedation, ataxia

Table 3
Summary of pharmacologic properties of antiepileptic drugs used as maintenance therapy in cats

Drug	Recommended Starting Oral Dose	Time to Steady-State Concentration (Days)	Reported Adverse Effects
Phenobarbital	1.5–2.5 mg/kg q 12 h	16	Sedation, ataxia Weight gain Blood dyscrasias Facial pruritis
Bromide	30 mg/kg q 24 h	37	Bronchial asthma Sedation Polydipsia Vomiting Weight gain
Gabapentin	5–10 mg/kg q 8–12 h	Not reported	Sedation, ataxia
Zonisamide	5 mg/kg q 12–24 h	7	Sedation, ataxia Anorexia Vomiting Diarrhea
Levetiracetam	20 mg/kg q 8 h	1	Sedation Inappetance Hypersalivation
Pregabalin	1–2 mg/kg q 12 h	Not reported	Sedation, ataxia

Pharmacokinetics

Phenobarbital is well absorbed after oral administration in dogs, with a reported bioavailability of approximately 90%[35,36] and an absorption half-life of approximately 1.3 hours.[36,37] Peak plasma concentrations are reached 4 to 8 hours after oral administration.[36] The elimination half-life of phenobarbital in normal dogs has been reported to range from 37 to 74 hours after multiple oral dosing.[37]

Phenobarbital undergoes hepatic metabolism, and is a potent inducer of cytochrome P450 (CYP) enzyme activity in the liver. Autoinduction can occur, whereby phenobarbital increases its own rate of metabolism over time. After 90 days of administration of phenobarbital to normal dogs at a daily oral dose of 5.5 mg/kg, the elimination half-life was shown to decrease from approximately 89 hours to 47 hours.[38]

Pharmacokinetic studies of phenobarbital in cats have demonstrated that peak concentrations are achieved approximately 1 to 1.5 hours after oral administration,[39] with an elimination half-life ranging from 43 to 76 hours.[39,40]

A parenteral form of phenobarbital is available for intramuscular or intravenous (IV) administration. The pharmacokinetics of intramuscular phenobarbital has not been explored in either dogs or cats, but studies in humans have demonstrated a similar absorption after intramuscular administration to that observed with oral administration.[41] The intramuscular route is useful for administering maintenance therapy in hospitalized patients that are unable to take oral medication. Elimination half-life in dogs after IV phenobarbital administration is approximately 93 hours.[35]

Clinical use

Phenobarbital is still considered by many practitioners to be the first-line drug for the treatment of epilepsy in both dogs and cats, based on its efficacy, low cost, ease of administration, and reasonable time required to achieve steady-state concentrations.

Available data suggest that phenobarbital is the most effective antiepileptic drug currently used in veterinary medicine. Open-label studies have shown phenobarbital to be effective in approximately 60% to 80% of epileptic dogs when plasma concentrations are maintained within the therapeutic range of 20 μg/mL to 45 μg/mL.[42,43] Furthermore, the superior efficacy of phenobarbital was demonstrated in a randomized controlled trial comparing phenobarbital to bromide as a first-line antiepileptic drug in dogs, in which 85% of dogs administered phenobarbital became seizure-free compared with 52% of dogs administered potassium bromide.[44] The recommended initial starting oral dose, 2.5 mg/kg to 3.0 mg/kg every 12 hours, is expected to achieve steady-state serum concentrations at the low end of the therapeutic range (20–25 μg/mL) in most dogs.[38] The recommended starting oral dose in cats of 1.5 mg/kg to 2.5 mg/kg every 12 hours is lower than that in dogs, as is the targeted serum concentrations of 15 μg/mL to 30 μg/mL.[45] Because of considerable variability in the pharmacokinetics of phenobarbital among individuals, serum drug concentrations should be measured approximately 2 weeks after initiating therapy to confirm that therapeutic levels have been reached. If the seizures are controlled on the current dose of phenobarbital, the animal should be evaluated at 6- to 12-month intervals, to screen for any adverse effects of the drug and to monitor for any changes in serum concentrations that might be of clinical relevance. The latter is particularly important with phenobarbital, because autoinduction can result in decreased serum concentrations over time. If seizures are not controlled, the phenobarbital dose should be increased by approximately 25% and serum concentrations reassessed in 2 weeks. This process is repeated as long as seizure control remains poor, until serum phenobarbital concentrations reach 30 μg/mL or intolerable side effects develop.

The timing of blood collections for phenobarbital monitoring is not important in most dogs, because the change in phenobarbital concentrations through a daily dosing interval is not therapeutically relevant.[46] Measurement of peak and trough samples should be performed, however, in dogs that continue to have seizures on phenobarbital therapy, to ensure that there is not a daily fluctuation in serum drug concentrations. In some instances, 3-times daily dosing might be indicated.

Phenobarbital can be administered IV as a treatment of acute repetitive seizures, although therapeutic effects can take as long as 30 minutes to achieve, because the drug is less lipid soluble than diazepam.[47] A loading dose of 12 mg/kg to 24 mg/kg IV has been recommended to achieve therapeutic concentrations rapidly.[47] In phenobarbital-naïve dogs, the author administers an initial dose of 12 mg/kg IV, followed by 2 mg/kg to 4 mg/kg increments every 20 to 30 minutes to effect, with a maximum dose of 24 mg/kg. For dogs on maintenance phenobarbital therapy and cats, the IV drug is initially given at 2 mg/kg to 4 mg/kg increments every 20 to 30 minutes to effect.

Adverse effects

Common adverse effects of phenobarbital include polydipsia, polyphagia, polyuria, lethargy, and ataxia and are seen in approximately half of dogs within the first month of initiating therapy.[44] In most dogs, these adverse effects tend to improve, if not resolve, over the course of several months.[44] Adverse effects reported in cats include sedation, ataxia, and weight gain.[48] Other, less common adverse effects described with phenobarbital administration include hyperexcitability[44] and movement disorders[49] in dogs, facial pruritis in cats,[48] and blood dyscrasias in both dogs and cats.[48,50] The latter is a rare, but potentially serious, idiosyncratic reaction to phenobarbital, in which any of the cell lines can be affected. Reported adverse effects are all reversible with discontinuation of phenobarbital therapy.

The adverse effect that tends to be of greatest concern is the potential for hepato-toxicity. It is common for dogs administered phenobarbital to have increases in serum liver–associated enzymes, notably alkaline phosphatase (ALP) and alanine amino-transferase (ALT), with no clinical evidence of liver disease.[51,52] The significance of the liver enzyme increases remain controversial. In a study by Müller and colleagues,[53] normal dogs were administered a daily oral 5-mg/kg dose of phenobarbital for 29 weeks and serially evaluated with laboratory analyses, abdominal imaging, and liver histopathology obtained with ultrasound-guided biopsy. Significant increases in ALT and ALP were noted, although no evidence of morphologic liver damage was observed histopathologically, leading the investigators to conclude that this likely is a reflection of enzyme induction rather than hepatic injury.[53] A more recent study eval-uated liver histopathology, as well as ALT and ALP activities, in liver homogenates from clinically healthy epileptic dogs that demonstrated elevations in serum liver–associated enzymes in conjunction with phenobarbital administration.[54] Compared with control dogs, phenobarbital-treated dogs did not have increased activities of ALT and ALP in liver homogenates but did demonstrate more severe and frequent his-topathologic abnormalities commonly associated with liver injury. Results from this study do not support enzyme induction as the cause for increases in serum ALT and ALP activities but rather suggest that they might reflect subclinical hepatic injury.

Nonetheless, clinical evidence of liver disease is uncommon with phenobarbital administration, and any changes are reversible with discontinuation of the drug if iden-tified early in the course of disease. To monitor for hepatic disease, laboratory ana-lyses performed at 6- to 12-month intervals should be evaluated for dramatic increases or decreases in serum-associated liver enzymes over time as well as any in-crease in phenobarbital serum concentration not associated with a concomitant dosage increase. In addition, monitoring of fasting serum bile acids, aspartate amino-transaminase, and bilirubin might be useful, because these values do not seem affected by the potential enzyme-inducing effects of phenobarbital.[53] Furthermore, a serum phenobarbital concentration of 30 μg/mL to 35 μg/mL should be considered the maximum acceptable level, because dogs with serum phenobarbital concentra-tions greater than 40 μg/mL seem at increased risk for hepatotoxicity.[55]

Phenobarbital administration can lower serum concentrations of free T_4 and total T_4 in dogs, but this is not associated with a hypothyroid state.[56–58] Consequently, clini-cians should use caution when interpreting the results of thyroid testing in dogs receiving phenobarbital, particularly if no clinical signs of hypothyroidism are present. In addition, phenobarbital alters the disposition of other drugs that undergo hepatic metabolism via the CYP system, including antiepileptic drugs, such as zonisamide[59] and diazepam.[60]

Phenobarbital has a narrow therapeutic index, although serious systemic side effects are uncommon. Routine, periodic patient monitoring enables most potential problems to be identified at an early stage. Furthermore, its established efficacy, ease of administration, and low cost offer clear advantages over other antiepileptic drugs, and phenobarbital is an important tool in the management of epilepsy in dogs and cats. A study designed to evaluate owners' perceptions regarding the care of epileptic dogs treated with phenobarbital discovered that most owners were pleased with their dog's quality of life on the medication.[61]

Bromide

Mechanism of action

Bromide is thought to exert its antiepileptic effect by hyperpolarizing the postsynaptic membrane.[62] After administration, bromide readily distributes to the extracellular space and then traverses the GABA-gated chloride channels in the postsynaptic membrane to accumulate intracellularly. Bromide crosses cell membranes faster than chloride due to its smaller hydrated diameter. The intracellular accumulation of bromide leads to membrane hyperpolarization.

Pharmacokinetics

The bioavailability of bromide after oral administration in normal dogs is approximately 46%.[63] Bromide is not bound to plasma proteins and can freely diffuse across cell membranes.[62] The elimination half-life ranges from 25 to 46 days in dogs[64]; accordingly, it can take several months to reach steady-state concentrations. The elimination half-life in cats is approximately 11 days.[64] No hepatic metabolism occurs, and bromide is excreted unchanged by the kidneys. Bromide undergoes tubular reabsorption in competition with chloride, such that changes in dietary chloride can alter the disposition of bromide.[65] A high dietary chloride load increases the excretion of bromide and shortens its half-life, whereas a low dietary chloride content slows the excretion of bromide and prolongs the half-life.

Clinical use

The anticonvulsive properties of bromide have been known since the mid-1800s, although its use in veterinary medicine has experienced a resurgence after a report in 1986 of the concurrent use of bromide and phenobarbital to control refractory epilepsy in dogs.[1] Bromide has not been approved by the US Food and Drug Administration for use in humans or animals. The product used in veterinary medicine is compounded into a solution, capsules, or tablets from either the potassium-derived or sodium-derived analytic grade chemical.

Bromide was originally described as an add-on treatment for epileptic dogs that were poorly controlled with phenobarbital and was reported to improve seizure control in 53% to 72% of dogs.[1,66,67] More recently, bromide has gained use as a sole antiepileptic therapy in dogs, either as a first-line drug or in dogs with intolerable side effects from phenobarbital.[44,67] A randomized controlled study comparing the safety and efficacy of bromide and phenobarbital as first-line antiepileptic therapy in dogs reported 52% of dogs became seizure-free on bromide.[44]

The recommended starting dose for potassium bromide is 30 mg/kg orally every 24 hours. Higher doses of 40 mg/kg to 80 mg/kg might be needed, however, when used as a sole antiepileptic agent. Therapeutic ranges have been reported as approximately 1.0 mg/mL to 2.0 mg/mL when administered in conjunction with phenobarbital and 1.0 mg/mL to 3.0 mg/mL when administered alone.[67] Because steady-state bromide concentrations are not achieved for several months, a loading dose of bromide can be administered at the initiation of treatment to achieve therapeutic concentrations of the drug more rapidly. A oral loading dose of 400 mg/kg to 600 mg/kg is recommended; this should be divided and administered with food. For rapid loading, the dose can be administered over 24 hours, whereas more gradual loading can be accomplished over 5 days. Although therapeutic serum levels can be obtained quicker by administering a loading dose, the time to reach steady-state concentrations is not altered.

The use of bromide has also been described in cats. An oral dose of 30 mg/kg/d has been shown to successfully control seizures in approximately 50% of cats treated.[64] The incidence of side effects is high, however, and consequently the routine use of bromide is not recommended in cats.

Adverse effects

Common adverse effects of bromide in dogs include vomiting, lethargy, ataxia, polyuria, polydipsia, and polyphagia.[44] Vomiting is presumably due to gastric irritation from the hypertonicity of the bromide salt. For this reason, it is recommended that bromide is administered with food. If vomiting persists, the daily dose can be divided into twice-daily administration, sodium bromide can be used instead of potassium bromide, or the compound can be encapsulated if the solution had been administered previously. The incidence of pancreatitis in dogs treated with a combination of phenobarbital and potassium bromide has been shown increased compared with dogs administered phenobarbital alone,[68] suggesting that bromide therapy might predispose to the development of pancreatitis. A causal relationship between the 2 has not been established, however. Efforts should be made to minimize changes in diet while on bromide therapy, because changes in dietary chloride can influence the rate of bromide excretion. If a diet change is necessary, the bromide level should be monitored closely for several months after the transition.

Signs of bromide toxicity in dogs develop in a dose-dependent manner and include alterations in consciousness, ataxia, and paresis that can be either upper motor neuron or lower motor neuron in character.[69] Clinical signs are most frequently recognized in dogs administered a total daily dose of bromide and serum bromide concentrations within the upper limit of the recommended ranges.[69] Treatment consisting of bromide dose reduction typically leads to rapid reversal of clinical signs. In severe cases, excretion of bromide can be facilitated by saline diuresis. Animals with renal impairment are at increased risk for the development of bromide toxicity and might require a reduction in initial dosage and more frequent monitoring of bromide levels.[70]

Adverse effects reported in cats include polydipsia, vomiting, weight gain, sedation, and coughing.[64] Coughing was reported in 38% of cats in one study[64] and is believed due to allergic bronchial disease. The respiratory compromise can be life-threatening and, for this reason, the use of bromide as an antiepileptic drug in cats is discouraged.

Gabapentin

Mechanism of action

The precise cellular mechanism of action of gabapentin is unclear. Despite being designed as a GABA agonist, it does not seem to act on the GABA receptor. There is evidence to suggest that much of the antiepileptic effect is due to binding to a specific modulatory protein of voltage-gated calcium channels, resulting in decreased release of excitatory neurotransmitters.[71]

Pharmacokinetics

Gabapentin is well absorbed after oral administration in dogs with maximum blood concentrations achieved within 2 hours.[72] Unlike humans and rodents, in which gabapentin is excreted unchanged in the urine, in dogs, approximately one-third of the absorbed dose undergoes liver metabolism prior to renal excretion,[72] with an elimination half-life of approximately 3 to 4 hours.[73] The pharmacokinetic properties of gabapentin in cats have not been described.

Clinical use

There are 2 published open-label trials evaluating the use of gabapentin as add-on therapy in dogs with refractory epilepsy. One study reported a positive response to therapy in 6 of 11 dogs,[74] whereas the other failed to identify a significant decrease in the number of seizures over the study period for the cohort of 17 dogs evaluated.[75] The recommended dose in dogs is 10 mg/kg to 20 mg/kg orally every 6 to 8 hours. Common side effects include sedation and ataxia. There are anecdotal reports of the use of gabapentin in epileptic cats, at a dose of 5 mg/kg to 10 mg/kg orally every 8 to 12 hours. The commercially available liquid formulation of gabapentin, which is often preferred when dosing cats and small dogs, contains xylitol (300 mg/mL).

Because of the potential for xylitol toxicity,[76] a tablet or capsule formulation of gabapentin should be preferentially used in dogs.

Zonisamide

Mechanism of action
Zonisamide is a sulfonamide drug with several pharmacologic effects that might contribute to its anticonvulsive properties. It has been demonstrated to block T-type calcium channels, inhibit voltage-gated sodium channels, enhance GABA release, and inhibit glutamate release.[77]

Pharmacokinetics
Zonisamide is well absorbed after oral administration to dogs, with a reported bioavailability of approximately 68% and maximum concentrations achieved in approximately 3 hours.[78] Elimination half-life is approximately 17 hours.[78] The majority of absorbed drug undergoes hepatic metabolism, followed by renal excretion.[78] Metabolism is believed to involve the CYP system, and concurrent administration of phenobarbital, which is a microsomal enzyme system inducer, has been shown to increase the clearance of zonisamide.[59] A pharmacokinetic study of zonisamide in cats demonstrated that maximum concentrations are achieved approximately 4 hours after oral administration, with an elimination half-life of approximately 33 hours.[79]

Clinical use
There is limited information on the efficacy of zonisamide in dogs, with 3 open-label trials published to date.[80–82] Two studies evaluated zonisamide as an add-on drug in a total of 25 dogs. Response rates of 58% to 82% were reported in these studies, with a median reduction in seizure frequency of 70% to 81%.[80,81] The third study evaluated zonisamide as monotherapy in 10 dogs, and reported a response rate of 60%.[82] The recommended starting dose in dogs is 5 mg/kg to 10 mg/kg orally every 12 hours. The high end of the dose range is needed when used in combination with phenobarbital, because concurrent phenobarbital administration increases the clearance of zonisamide.[59] Adverse effects described in dogs include sedation, ataxia, and loss of appetite.[80–82] In addition, recent reports suggest that more serious adverse effects can occur infrequently with zonisamide administration, including hepatotoxicity[83,84] and renal tubular acidosis.[85] There are anecdotal reports of the use of zonisamide in cats, with oral doses of 5 mg/kg orally every 12 to 24 hours most commonly used. A toxicity study in normal cats demonstrated, however, that a daily oral dose of 20 mg/kg resulted in adverse effects in half of the cats, including anorexia, diarrhea, vomiting, lethargy, and ataxia.[79]

Because zonisamide has a wide therapeutic index, serum concentrations are not routinely measured. A therapeutic range has not been established in either dogs or cats, although the human therapeutic range of 10 μg/mL to 40 μg/mL has been extrapolated for use in dogs.[80] The author finds it useful to measure serum concentrations when satisfactory seizure control is not obtained, to determine whether a dosage increase might be warranted.

Levetiracetam

Mechanism of action
Levetiracetam is unique among antiepileptic drugs with respect to its mechanism of action, in that it modulates the release of neurotransmitters by selective binding to the presynaptic protein SVA2.[86] The exact mechanism by which this produces its antiepileptic effect, however, is poorly understood. Levetiracetam has been shown to reduce current through voltage-gated calcium channels, inhibit release of calcium

from intraneuronal calcium stores, and inhibit burst firing of neurons, thereby suppressing hypersynchronization and propagation of seizure activity.[87]

Pharmacokinetics

Levetiracetam is well absorbed after oral administration in dogs, with a bioavailability of 100%.[88] Absorption is rapid, with peak concentrations achieved in less than 2 hours.[88,89] The drug is primarily excreted unchanged in the urine of dogs,[90] with an elimination half-life of 3 to 6 hours.[88–91] Although levetiracetam is not metabolized by the liver, concurrent administration of phenobarbital has been shown to increase its clearance, perhaps by inducing its oxidative metabolism in extrahepatic tissues.[92] A pharmacokinetic study in cats demonstrated an oral bioavailability of 100%, with maximum concentrations reached in approximately 1.7 hours and an elimination half-life of approximately 3 hours.[93]

Clinical use

An open-label study evaluating the efficacy of levetiracetam as an add-on treatment in 14 dogs refractory to phenobarbital and bromide documented a response rate of 57%.[94] The efficacy of levetiracetam as add-on therapy was further evaluated in a randomized clinical trial involving 34 dogs with refractory epilepsy.[95] A significant decrease in seizure frequency compared to baseline was observed in levetiracetam-treated dogs; however, no significant change in seizure frequency was identified when levetiracetam treatment was compared with placebo.[95] The use of levetiracetam has also been described in cats, with 7 of 10 cats reported to have a favorable response to treatment.[96]

The recommended dose in both dogs and cats is 20 mg/kg orally every 8 hours. An extended release formulation of the drug is also available, and a pharmacokinetic study supports its use in dogs with a 12-hour dosing interval.[97] Common adverse effects in dogs include sedation and ataxia.[94,95] Lethargy, inappetence, and hypersalivation have been described in cats.[93,96]

A parenteral form of levetiracetam is available for the emergency treatment of seizures. A recent, randomized controlled trial involving 19 dogs demonstrated that IV levetiracetam administered at a dose of 30 mg/kg to 60 mg/kg was safe and potentially effective for the treatment of status epilepticus in dogs.[98]

Pregabalin

Mechanism of action

Pregabalin is a newer-generation drug in the same class as gabapentin. The mechanism of action is similar to gabapentin, although pregabalin has a greater affinity for the binding site by which the drugs exert their effect and consequently has a greater potency than gabapentin.[71]

Pharmacokinetics

A single pharmacokinetic study on oral administration of pregabalin in normal dogs demonstrated that maximum concentrations are achieved at 1.5 hours and an elimination half-life of approximately 7 hours.[99]

Clinical use

There is a single, published, open-label study on the use of pregabalin in dogs with refractory epilepsy, in which 7 of 11 dogs were classified as having a positive response to treatment.[100] The recommended dose for dogs is 3 mg/kg to 4 mg/kg orally every 8 hours; however, in order to minimize side effects, it is suggested that treatment be initiated at 2 mg/kg and the dose increased by 1 mg/kg each week until the target dose is reached. Common side effects include sedation and ataxia. There are anecdotal reports of the use of pregabalin in cats, with a dose of 1 mg/kg to 2 mg/kg orally every 12 hours most commonly mentioned.

NONPHARMACOLOGIC TREATMENT OPTIONS
Vagal Nerve Stimulation

Alternative, nonmedical methods of seizure control have been explored for patients with epilepsy who experience poor control with antiepileptic medication. One alternative therapy that has proved successful in humans is vagal nerve stimulation. This form of treatment involves the surgical implantation of a pacemaker-type device that delivers repetitive electrical stimulation to the vagus nerve in the neck. A randomized controlled study evaluated vagal nerve stimulation in 10 dogs with refractory epilepsy and found the treatment to be potentially safe and efficacious in some dogs.[101] Due to the expense of the device and the inability to predict whether or not an individual animal will respond, however, this form of therapy is rarely used in veterinary medicine.

Dietary Modification

Dietary modification is another form of nonpharmacologic therapy that has been advocated in the treatment of epilepsy. The ketogenic diet has been used successfully to control seizures in children, and consists of a stringent high-fat, low-carbohydrate, low-protein diet. A randomized controlled study was undertaken to evaluate a ketogenic diet as a treatment for 12 dogs with epilepsy, and no beneficial effect was identified.[102] Other dietary modifications that have been evaluated in dogs include a hypoallergenic diet and fatty acid supplementation. An abstract reporting on a retrospective evaluation of the use of hypoallergenic diet in dogs with poorly controlled seizures described improved seizure control in 7 of 8 dogs, although the full results of this study have not been published in a peer-reviewed source.[103] A randomized controlled trial evaluating the use of essential fatty acid supplementation in 15 dogs with refractory epilepsy found no significant difference in seizure frequency between fatty acid supplementation and placebo.[104] Additional studies are warranted to further explore the potential role of dietary modification in the treatment of epilepsy.

ACUTE MANAGEMENT OF SEIZURES AT HOME

Dogs with poorly controlled seizures place a significant financial and emotional burden on their owners, especially if frequent veterinary visits to obtain emergency care are required. Consequently, the successful management of an epileptic dog should include recommendations for emergency care of seizures at home.

Rectal administration of the parenteral formulation of diazepam has been used most frequently in this regard and has been shown to decrease the number of cluster seizure events over a 24-hour period.[105] The recommended dose is 1 mg/kg of diazepam administered at the onset of seizures, given up to 3 times over a 24-hour period. Dogs receiving phenobarbital should be administered a dose of 2 mg/kg, because chronic phenobarbital therapy reduces peak benzodiazepine concentrations after the administration of rectal diazepam.[60] Diazepam is inactivated by light and adheres to plastic, so the parenteral formulation of the drug should be dispensed in the original glass vial with instructions for the owner to draw up the required amount with a needle and syringe when needed. The needle is then removed, and a rubber catheter or teat cannula is placed on the syringe for rectal administration. Suppository forms of the drug are commercially available, but the pharmacokinetics of these products has not been evaluated in dogs. A recent pharmacokinetic study evaluating a

Table 4
Dose and route of administration for benzodiazepines in the acute management of seizures at home

Drug	Dose	Routes of Administration	References
Diazepam	0.5–1.0 mg/kg	Rectal, intranasal	105,107,108
Midazolam	0.2–0.5 mg/kg	Intranasal, intramuscular[a]	109,110
Lorazepam	0.2 mg/kg	Intranasal[a]	111

[a] Pharmacokinetic studies do not support the administration of either midazolam[110] or lorazepam[112] by the rectal route.

compounded diazepam rectal suppository in dogs demonstated that presumed therapeutic plasma concentrations of diazepam or its active metabolite nordiazepam were not achieved within an acceptable time frame to be effective as emergency treatment for seizures at home.[106]

The parenteral form of diazepam has periodically been unavailable, prompting the need to dispense other benzodiazepines, such as midazolam or lorazepam, for home use. Recommendations of the dose and route of administration are based on pharmacokinetic studies in dogs (Table 4), although there are no studies evaluating the efficacy of such treatment in dogs with seizures.

Additional doses of maintenance oral antiepileptic drugs, or pulse therapy with one of the newer drugs, have also been advocated to treat cluster seizures at home, but there are no published reports documenting this use.

REFERENCES

1. Schwartz-Porsche D. Epidemiological, clinical and pharmacokinetic studies in spontaneously epileptic dogs and cats. Proceedings of the 4th Annual American College of Veterinary Internal Medicine Forum, Washington, DC. 1986, 11-61-11-63.
2. Bunch SE. Anticonvulsant drug therapy in companion animals. In: Kirk RW, editor. Current Veterinary Therapy IX. Philadelphia: WB Saunders Co; 1986. p. 836–44.
3. Pakozdy A, Leschnik M, Sarchahi AA, et al. Clinical comparison of primary versus secondary epilepsy in 125 cats. J Feline Med Surg 2010;12:910–6.
4. McNamara JD. Drugs effective in the therapy of epilepsies. In: Hardman JG, Limbird LE, editors. Goodman and Gilman's the pharmacologic basis of therapeutics. New York: McGraw-Hill; 1996. p. 461–85.
5. Berg AT, Berkovic SF, Brodie MJ, et al. Revised terminology and concepts for organization of seizures and epilepsies: report of the ILAE Commission on Classification and Terminology, 2005-2009. Epilepsia 2010;51:676–85.
6. Weissl J, Hülsmeyer V, Brauer C, et al. Disease progression and treatment response of idiopathic epilepsy in Australian shepherd dogs. J Vet Intern Med 2012;26:116–25.
7. Bielfeft SW, Redman HC, McClellan RO. Sire- and sex-related differences in rates of epileptiform seizures in a purebred Beagle dog colony. Am J Vet Res 1971;32:2039–48.
8. Famula TR, Oberhauer AM. Segregation analysis of epilepsy in the Belgian Tervueren dog. Vet Rec 2000;147:218–21.
9. Kathmann I, Jaggy A, Busato A, et al. Clinical and genetic investigations of idiopathic epilepsy in the Bernese Mountain dog. J Small Anim Pract 1999;40: 319–25.

10. Hülsmeyer V, Zimmermann R, Brauer C, et al. Epilepsy in Border collies: clinical manifestation, outcome and mode of inheritance. J Vet Intern Med 2010;24: 171–8.
11. Lohi H, Young EJ, Fitzmaurice SN, et al. Expanded repeat in canine epilepsy. Science 2005;307:81.
12. Licht BG, Licht MH, Harper KM, et al. Clinical presentation of naturally occurring canine seizures: similarities to human seizures. Epilepsy Behav 2002;3:460–70.
13. Patterson EE, Armstrong JP, O'Brien DR, et al. Clinical description and mode of inheritance of idiopathic epilepsy in English Springer Spaniels. J Am Vet Med Assoc 2005;226:54–8.
14. Falco MJ, Barker J, Wallace ME. The genetics of epilepsy in the British Alsatian. J Small Anim Pract 1974;15:685–92.
15. Srenk P, Jaggy A. Interictal electroencephalographic findings in a family of Golden Retrievers with idiopathic epilepsy. J Small Anim Pract 1996;37:317–21.
16. Casal ML, Munuve RM, Janis MA, et al. Epilepsy in Irish Wolfhounds. J Vet Intern Med 2006;20:131–5.
17. Hall SJ, Wallace ME. Canine epilepsy: a genetic counseling programme for Keeshounds. Vet Rec 1996;138:358–60.
18. Jaggy A, Faissler D, Gaillard C, et al. Genetic aspects of idiopathic epilepsy in Labrador Retrievers. J Small Anim Pract 1998;39:275–80.
19. Jokinen TS, Metsähonkala L, Bergamasco L, et al. Benign familial juvenile epilepsy in Lagotto Romagnolo dogs. J Vet Intern Med 2007;21:464–71.
20. Morita T, Shimada A, Takeuchi T, et al. Cliniconeuropathologic findings of familial frontal lobe epilepsy in Shetland Sheepdogs. Can J Vet Res 2002;66:35–41.
21. Licht BG, Lin S, Luo Y, et al. Clinical characteristics and mode of inheritance of familial focal seizures in Standard Poodles. J Am Vet Med Assoc 2007;231: 1520–8.
22. Patterson EE, Mickelson JD, Da Y, et al. Clinical characteristics and inheritance of idiopathic epilepsy in Vizslas. J Vet Intern Med 2003;17:319–25.
23. Heynold Y, Faissler D, Steffen F, et al. Clinical, epidemiological and treatment results of idiopathic epilepsy in 54 Labrador retrievers: a long-term study. J Small Anim Pract 1997;38:7–14.
24. Kwan P, Brodie MJ. Early identification of refractory epilepsy. N Engl J Med 2000;342:314–9.
25. Jull P, DeRisio L, Horton C, et al. Effect of prolonged status epilepticus as a result of intoxication on epileptogenesis in a UK canine population. Vet Rec 2011;169:361–4.
26. Shovron S, Luciano AL. Prognosis of chronic and newly diagnosed epilepsy: revisiting temporal aspects. Curr Opin Neurol 2007;20:208–12.
27. Rogawski MA, Johsnon MR. Intrinsic severity as a determinant of antiepileptic drug refractoriness. Epilepsy Curr 2008;8:127–30.
28. Muñana KR, Nettifee-Osborne JA, Bergman RL, et al. Association between ABCB 1 genotype and seizure outcome in Collies with epilepsy. J Vet Intern Med 2012;26:1358–64.
29. Leppik IE. Monotherapy and polytherapy. Neurology 2000;55:S25–9.
30. Muñana KR, Zhang D, Patterson EE. Placebo effect in canine epilepsy trials. J Vet Intern Med 2010;24:166–70.
31. Podell M. Seizures in dogs. Vet Clin North Am Small Anim Pract 1996;26: 779–810.
32. Berendt M, Gredal H, Kjaer Ersboll A, et al. Premature death, risk factors, and life patterns in dogs with epilepsy. J Vet Intern Med 2007;21:754–9.

33. Twyman RE, Rogers CJ, Macdonald RL. Differential regulation of gamma-aminobutyric acid receptor channels by diazepam and phenobarbital. Ann Neurol 1989;25:213–20.
34. Heyer E, Macdonald R. Barbiturate reduction of calcium-dependent action potentials: correlation with anesthetic action. Brain Res 1982;236:157–71.
35. Pedersoli WM, Wike JS, Ravis WR. Pharmacokinetics of single doses of pheno-barbital given intravenously and orally to dogs. Am J Vet Res 1987;48:679–83.
36. Al-Tahan F, Frey HH. Absorption kinetics and bioavailability of phenobarbital after oral administration to dogs. J Vet Pharmacol Ther 1985;8:205–7.
37. Ravis WR, Nachreiner RF, Pedersoli WM, et al. Pharmacokinetics of phenobar-bital in dogs after multiple oral administration. Am J Vet Res 1984;45:1283–6.
38. Ravis WR, Pedersoli WM, Wike JS. Pharmacokinetics of phenobarbital in dogs given multiple doses. Am J Vet Res 1989;50:1343–7.
39. Cochrane SM, Black WD, Parent JM, et al. Pharmacokinetics of phenobarbital in the cat following intravenous and oral administration. Can J Vet Res 1990;54: 132–8.
40. Cochrane SM, Parent JM, Black WD, et al. Pharmacokinetics of phenobarbital in the cat following multiple oral administration. Can J Vet Res 1990;54:309–12.
41. Wilensky A, Friel P, Levy R, et al. Pharmacokinetics of phenobarbital in normal subjects and epileptic patients. Eur J Clin Pharmacol 1982;23:87–92.
42. Schwartz-Porsche D, Loscher W, Frey HH. Therapeutic efficacy of phenobar-bital and primidone in canine epilepsy: a comparison. J Vet Pharmacol Ther 1985;8:113–9.
43. Farnbach GC. Serum concentrations and efficacy of phenytoin, phenobarbital, and primidone in canine epilepsy. J Am Vet Med Assoc 1984;184:1117–20.
44. Boothe DM, Dewey C, Carpenter DM. Comparison of phenobarbital with bro-mide as a first-choice antiepileptic drug for treatment of epilepsy in dogs. J Am Vet Med Assoc 2012;240:1073–83.
45. Schwartz-Porsche D, Kaiser E. Feline epilepsy. Probl Vet Med 1989;1:629–49.
46. Levitski RE, Trepanier LA. Effect of timing of blood collection on serum pheno-barbital concentrations in dogs with epilepsy. J Am Vet Med Assoc 2000;217: 200–4.
47. Boothe DM. Anticonvulsant therapy in small animals. Vet Clin North Am Small Anim Pract 1998;28:411–48.
48. Quesnel AE, Parent JM, McDonell W. Clinical management and outcome of cats with seizure disorders: 30 cases (1991-1993). J Am Vet Med Assoc 1997;210: 72–7.
49. Kube SA, Vernau KM, LeCouteur RA. Dyskinesia associated with oral phenobar-bital administration in a dog. J Vet Intern Med 2006;20:1238–40.
50. Jacobs G, Calvert C, Kaufman A. Neutropenia and thrombocytopenia in three dogs treated with anticonvulsants. J Am Vet Med Assoc 1998;212:681–4.
51. Chauvet AE, Feldman EC, Kass PH. Effects of phenobarbital administration on results of serum biochemical analyses and adrenocortical function tests in epileptic dogs. J Am Vet Med Assoc 1995;207:1305–7.
52. Foster SF, Church DB, Watson ADJ. Effects of phenobarbitone on serum biochemical tests in dogs. Aust Vet J 2001;78:23–6.
53. Müller PB, Taboada J, Hosgood G, et al. Effects of long-term phenobarbital treatment on the liver in dogs. J Vet Intern Med 2000;14:165–71.
54. Gaskill CL, Miller LM, Mattoon JS, et al. Liver histopathology and liver and serum alanine aminotransferase and alkaline phosphatase activities in epileptic dogs receiving phenobarbital. Vet Pathol 2005;42:147–60.

55. Dayrell-Hart B, Steinberg SA, VanWinkle TJ, et al. Hepatotoxicity of phenobarbital in dogs: 18 cases (1985-1989). J Am Vet Med Assoc 1991;199:1060–6.
56. Kantrowitz LB, Peterson ME, Trepanier LA, et al. Serum total thyroxine, total triiodothyronine, free thyroxine, and thyrotropin concentrations in epileptic dogs treated with anticonvulsants. J Am Vet Med Assoc 1999;214:1804–8.
57. Gaskill CL, Burton SA, Gelens HC, et al. Effects of phenobarbital treatment on serum thyroxine and thyroid-stimulating hormone concentrations in epileptic dogs. J Am Vet Med Assoc 1999;215:489–96.
58. Müller PB, Wolfsheimer KJ, Taboada J, et al. Effects of long-term phenobarbital treatment on the thyroid and adrenal axis and adrenal function tests in dogs. J Vet Intern Med 2000;14:157–63.
59. Orito K, Saito M, Fukunaga K, et al. Pharmacokinetics of zonisamide and drug interaction with phenobarbital in dogs. J Vet Pharmacol Ther 2008;31:259–64.
60. Wagner SO, Sams RA, Podell M. Chronic phenobarbital therapy reduces plasma benzodiazepine concentrations after intravenous and rectal administration of diazepam in the dog. J Vet Pharmacol Ther 1998;21:335–41.
61. Lord LK, Podell M. Owner perception of the care of long-term phenobarbital-treated epileptic dogs. J Small Anim Pract 1999;40:11–5.
62. Uthman BM. Less commonly used antiepileptic drugs. In: Wyllie E, Casciano GD, Gidal BE, et al, editors. Wyllie's treatment of epilepsy Principles and practice. 5th edition. Philadelphia: Lippincott Williams & Wilkins; 2011. p. 779–89.
63. Trepanier LA, Babish JG. Pharmacokinetic properties of bromide in dogs after the intravenous and oral administration of single doses. Res Vet Sci 1995;58:248–51.
64. Boothe DM, George KL, Couch P. Disposition and clinical use of bromide in cats. J Vet Med Assoc 2002;221:1131–5.
65. Trepanier LA, Babish JG. Effect of dietary chloride content on bromide elimination and dosage in dogs. Res Vet Sci 1995;58:252–5.
66. Podell M, Fenner WR. Bromide therapy in refractory canine idiopathic epilepsy. J Vet Intern Med 1993;7:318–27.
67. Trepanier LA, Van Schoick A, Schwark WS, et al. Therapeutic serum drug concentrations in epileptic dogs treated with potassium bromide alone or in combination with other anticonvulsants: 122 cases (1992-1996). J Am Vet Med Assoc 1998;213:1449–53.
68. Gaskill CL, Cribb AE. Pancreatitis associated with potassium bromide/phenobarbital combination therapy in epileptic dogs. Can Vet J 2000;41:555–8.
69. Rossmeisl JH, Inzana KD. Clinical signs, risk factors, and outcomes associated with bromide toxicosis (bromism) in dogs with idiopathic epilepsy. J Am Vet Med Assoc 2009;234:1425–31.
70. Nichols EF, Trepanier LA, Linn K. Bromide toxicosis secondary to renal insufficiency in an epileptic dog. J Am Vet Med Assoc 1996;208:231–3.
71. Sills GJ. The mechanism of action of gabapentin and pregabalin. Curr Opin Pharmacol 2006;6:108–13.
72. Radulovic LL, Türck D, Von Hodenberg A, et al. Disposition of gabapentin (Neurontin) in mice, rats, dogs and monkeys. Drug Metab Dispos 1995;23:441–8.
73. Vollmer KO, von Hodenberg A, Kölle EU. Pharmacokinetics and metabolism of gabapentin in rat, dog and man. Arzneimittelforschung 1986;36:830–9.
74. Platt SR, Adams V, Garosi LS, et al. Treatment with gabapentin of 11 dogs with refractory idiopathic epilepsy. Vet Rec 2006;159:881–4.

75. Govendir M, Perkins M, Malik R. Improving seizure control in dogs with refractory epilepsy using gabapentin as an adjunctive agent. Aust Vet J 2005;83: 602–8.

76. Dunayer EK, Gwaltnew-Brant SM. Acute hepatic failure and coagulopathy associated with xylitol ingestion in eight dogs. J Am Vet Med Assoc 2006;229: 1113–7.

77. Holder JL Jr, Wilfond AA. Zonisamide in the treatment of epilepsy. Expert Opin Pharmacother 2011;12:2573–81.

78. Boothe DM, Perkins J. Disposition and safety of zonisamide after intravenous and oral single dose and oral multiple dosing in normal hound dogs. J Vet Pharmacol Ther 2008;31:544–53.

79. Hasegawa D, Kobayashi M, Kuwabara T, et al. Pharmacokinetics and toxicity of zonisamide in cats. J Feline Med Surg 2008;10:418–21.

80. Dewey CW, Guiliano R, Boothe DW, et al. Zonisamide therapy for refractory idiopathic epilepsy in dogs. J Am Anim Hosp Assoc 2004;40:285–91.

81. von Klopmann T, Rambeck B, Tipold A. Prospective study of zonisamide therapy for refractory idiopathic epilepsy in dogs. J Small Anim Pract 2007;48:134–8.

82. Chung JY, Hwang CY, Chae JS, et al. Zonisamide monotherpy for idiopathic epilepsy in dogs. N Z Vet J 2012;60:357–9.

83. Miller ML, Center SA, Randolph JF, et al. Apparent acute idiosyncratic hepatic necrosis associated with zonisamide administration in a dog. J Vet Intern Med 2011;25:1156–60.

84. Schwartz M, Muñana KR, Olby NJ. Possible drug-induced hepatopathy in a dog receiving zonisamide monotherapy for treatment of cryptogenic epilepsy. J Vet Med Sci 2011;73:1505–8.

85. Cook AK, Allen AK, Espinosa D, et al. Renal tubular acidosis associated with zonisamide therapy in a dog. J Vet Intern med 2011;25:1454–7.

86. Lynch BA, Lamberg N, Nocka K, et al. The synaptic vesicle protein SVA2 is the binding site for the antiepileptic drug LEV. Proc Natl Acad Sci 2004;101: 9861–6.

87. Surges R, Volynski KE, Walker MC. Is levetiracetam different from other antiepileptic drugs? Levetiracetam and its cellular mechanism of action in epilepsy revisited. Ther Adv Neurol Disord 2008;1:13–24.

88. Patterson EE, Goel V, Cloyd JC, et al. Intramuscular, intravenous and oral levetiracetam in dogs: safety and pharmacokinetics. J Vet Pharmacol Ther 2008;31: 253–8.

89. Moore SA, Muñana KR, Papich MG, et al. Levetiracetam pharmacokinetics in healthy dogs following oral administration of single and multiple doses. Am J Vet Res 2010;71:337–41.

90. Isoherranen N, Yagen B, Soback S, et al. Pharmacokinetics of levetiracetam and its enantiomer (R)-alpha-ethyl-2-oxo-pyrrolidine acetamide in dogs. Epilepsia 2001;42:825–30.

91. Dewey CW, Bailey KS, Boothe DM, et al. Pharmacokinetics of single-dose intravenous levetiracetam administration in normal dogs. J Vet Emerg Crit Care 2008;18:153–7.

92. Moore SA, Muñana KR, Papich MG, et al. The pharmacokinetics of levetiracetam in healthy dogs concurrently receiving phenobarbital. J Vet Pharmacol Ther 2010;34:31–4.

93. Carnes MB, Axlund TW, Boothe DM. Pharmacokinetics of levetiracetam after oral and intravenous administration of a single dose to clinically normal cats. Am J Vet Res 2011;72:1247–52.

94. Volk HA, Matiasek LA, Luján Feliu-Pascual A, et al. The efficacy and tolerability of levetiracetam in pharmacoresistant epileptic dogs. Vet J 2008;176:310–9.
95. Muñana KR, Thomas WB, Inzana KD, et al. Evaluation of levetiracetam as adjunctive treatment for refractory canine epilepsy: a randomized, placebo-controlled crossover trial. J Vet Intern Med 2012;26:341–8.
96. Bailey KS, Dewey CW, Boothe DM, et al. Levetiracetam as an adjunct to pheno-barbital treatment in cats with suspected idiopathic epilepsy. J Am Vet Med Assoc 2008;232:867–72.
97. Beasley MJ, Boothe DM. The pharmacokinetics of single dose extended release Keppra® with and without food in healthy adult dogs [abstract]. J Vet Intern Med 2012;26:819.
98. Hardy BT, Patterson EE, Cloyd JM, et al. Double-masked, placebo-controlled study of intravenous levetiracetam for the treatment of status epilepticus and acute repetitive seizures in dogs. J Vet Intern Med 2012;26:334–40.
99. Salazar V, Dewey CW, Schwark W, et al. Pharmacokinetics of single-dose oral pregabalin administration in normal dogs. Vet Anaesth Analg 2009;36:574–80.
100. Dewey CW, Cerda-Gonzalz S, Levine JM, et al. Pregabalin as an adjunct to phenobarbital, potassium bromide, or a combination of phenobarbital and po-tassium bromide for treatment of dogs with suspected idiopathic epilepsy. J Am Vet Med Assoc 2009;235:1442–9.
101. Muñana KR, Vitek SM, Tarver WB, et al. Use of vagal nerve stimulation as a treat-ment for refractory epilepsy in dogs. J Am Vet Med Assoc 2002;221:977–83.
102. Patterson EE, Muñana KR, Kirk CA, et al. Results of a ketogenic food trial for dogs with idiopathic epilepsy [abstract]. J Vet Intern Med 2005;19:421.
103. Luján A, Scott SD, Anderson TJ. The role of diet in refractory canine epilepsy - a retrospective case series [abstract]. In: BSAVA Congress 2004: Scientific Proceedings. Quedgeley, UK: British Small Animal Veterinary Association; 2004. p. 53.
104. Matthews H, Granger N, Wood J, et al. Effects of essential fatty acid supplemen-tation in dogs with idiopathic epilepsy: a clinical trial. Vet J 2012;191:396–8.
105. Podell M. The use of diazepam per rectum at home for the acute management of cluster seizures in dogs. J Vet Intern Med 1995;8:68–74.
106. Probst CW, Thomas WB, Moyers TD, et al. Evaluation of plasma diazepam and nordiazepam concentrations following administration of diazepam intravenously or via suppository per rectum in dogs. Am J Vet Res 2013;74:611–5.
107. Platt SR, Scott KC, Chrisman CL, et al. Comparison of plasma benzodiazepine concentrations following intranasal and intravenous administration of diazepam to dogs. Am J Vet Res 2000;61:651–4.
108. Musulin SE, Mariani CL, Papich MG. Diazepam pharmacokinetics after nasal drop and atomized nasal administration in dogs. J Vet Pharmacol Ther 2011; 34:17–24.
109. Eagleson JS, Platt SR, Elder Strong DL, et al. Bioavailability of a novel midazo-lam gel after intranasal administration in dogs. Am J Vet Res 2012;73:539–45.
110. Schwartz M, Muñana KR, Nettifee-Osborne JA, et al. The pharmacokinetics of midazolam after intravenous, intramuscular, and rectal administration in healthy dogs. J Vet Pharmacol Ther 2012 Dec 19 [Epub ahead of print].
111. Mariani CL, Clemmons RM, Lee-Ambrose L, et al. A comparison of intranasal and intravenous lorazepam in normal dogs [abstract]. J Vet Intern Med 2003;17:402.
112. Podell M, Wagner SO, Sams RA. Lorazepam concentrations in plasma following its intravenous and rectal administration in dogs. J Vet Pharmacol Ther 1998;21: 158–60.

Update on Immununosuppressive Therapies for Dogs and Cats

Katrina R. Viviano, DVM, PhD

KEYWORDS

- Glucocorticoids • Cyclosporine • Azathioprine • Chlorambucil • Vincristine
- Human immunoglobulin • Mycophenolate • Leflunomide

KEY POINTS

- Understand mechanisms of action, adverse effects, and the clinical limitations of the common drugs (glucocorticoids [GCs], cyclosporine, azathioprine, and chlorambucil) used in the long-term management of immune-mediated diseases.
- Appreciate the clinical situations in which the use of human intravenous immunoglobulin (hIVIG) versus vincristine is most appropriate.
- Recognize the advantages and disadvantages of using mycophenolate and leflunomide in the treatment of immune-mediated disease in dogs and cats.

INTRODUCTION

The body's immune system is essential for protecting it from a variety of pathogens and other external insults. It is through the complex interactions between the cells and mediators of both the innate and adaptive immune systems that the immune system is tightly regulated and homeostasis is established. Autoimmune diseases arise from dysregulation of either the innate or adaptive immune system or both.[1] The complexity of immune dysregulation is not well understood but is likely multifactoral, including inherent genetic factors and/or environmental triggers (ie, infectious agents, drugs, vaccines, or neoplasia). In some patients, the immune system may be appropriately or inappropriately triggered, subsequently leading to lymphocyte dysfunction, for example, failure of lymphocyte selection and/or the generation of antibodies or T cells directed toward self-antigens.[2] The inappropriately stimulated immune system produces a marked local or systemic inflammatory response leading to tissue destruction and clinical disease.

Disclosures: The author has nothing to disclose.
Department of Medical Sciences, School of Veterinary Medicine, University of Wisconsin, 2015 Linden Drive, Madison, WI, USA
E-mail address: viviano@svm.vetmed.wisc.edu

Some of the more common systemic inflammatory diseases with an autoimmune cause in dogs and cats include protein-losing enteropathy/inflammatory bowel disease, immune-mediated hemolytic anemia, immune-mediated thrombocytopenia (IMT), immune-mediated polyarthritis, and feline asthma.[3] Despite the varying and incompletely understood pathogenic mechanisms or triggers among this group of diseases, immune dysfunction is central to tissue injury and the rationale for use of immunomodulatory therapies. The focus of this article is to provide an update on some of the more common immunosuppressive therapies used in small animal veterinary medicine. Few of these immunosuppressive drugs or protocols are well studied in veterinary species but their use has been adapted or extrapolated from human medicine in the treatment of autoimmune diseases or in the management of organ transplantation. The goals of therapy are to induce disease remission through the inhibition of inflammation and the modulation of lymphocyte function.

FIRST-LINE AND SECOND-LINE IMMUNOSUPPRESSIVE DRUGS
Glucocorticoids

Proposed mechanism
GCs affect most, if not all, cells of the body through their binding to the intracellular cytoplasmic GC receptor.[4,5] Once the GC-receptor complex is translocated to the nucleus, it binds DNA GC response elements influencing gene transcription.[6] The cellular effects of GCs are considered dose dependent. At antiinflammatory doses, GCs inhibit phospholipase A2 and the release of proinflammatory cytokines as well as stabilize granulocyte cell membranes. At immunosuppressive doses, GCs target macrophage function by down regulating Fc receptor expression, decreasing responsiveness to antibody-sensitized cell and decreasing antigen processing.[7–10] GCs suppress T-cell function and induce apoptosis of T cells and with chronic use B-cell antibody production may be inhibited in some patients.[5,11]

Adverse effects/drug interactions
The wide cellular/tissue distribution of the GC receptor makes significant systemic effects unavoidable.[12] Adverse effects include iatrogenic hyperadrenocorticism, adrenal gland suppression, gastrointestinal ulceration, insulin resistance and secondary diabetes mellitus, muscle catabolism, delayed wound healing, opportunistic infections, and behavior changes. Clinical signs of hyperadrenocorticism are more common in dogs and include polydipsia, polyuria, polyphagia, weight gain, and increased panting. In addition, some dogs experience elevations in serum alkaline phosphatase activity secondary to the induction of the steroid-induced isoenzyme. The coadministration of GC with nonsteroidal antiinflammatory drugs is contraindicated due to the significant risk of gastrointestinal ulceration or perforation.[13]

Clinical use
Despite the long list of clinically significant adverse effects associated with either short-duration high-dose or chronic low-dose GC therapy, GCs remain the mainstay or first-line therapy in the treatment of inflammatory and autoimmune diseases in dogs and cats (e.g. immune-mediated anemia, IMT, immune-mediated polyarthritis, inflammatory bowel disease, and feline asthma). Advantages of GCs are their systemic impact on both innate and acquired immunity and their relative rapid onset of action, thereby maintaining their role in the acute management of inflammatory/immune-mediated diseases. The goal of therapy is to achieve clinical remission and slowly taper the dose of GCs to the lowest dose that controls the inflammatory or immune-mediated disease targeted. On a case-by-case basis, GCs may be used in combination

with other immunosuppressive agents in the treatment of inflammatory or immune-mediated diseases in dogs and cats, especially in patients that are nonresponsive to GCs alone or present with severe life-threatening disease.

Pharmacokinetics/pharmaceutics

Available GCs vary in their potency, route of administration, and duration of action (**Table 1**).[14] The most common intermediate-acting systemic GCs used in veterinary medicine include prednisone/prednisolone. Prednisone is a prodrug that is metabolized to its active form prednisolone. Cats are reported to achieve higher plasma concentrations (4–5 times higher area under the curve) when administered oral prednisolone versus prednisone,[15] suggesting cats either have lower prednisone absorption and/or decreased prednisone conversion to prednisolone.

Alternative forms of GCs should be considered in specific patient populations. In patients with severe malabsorption, injectable dexamethasone sodium phosphate may provide improved bioavailability as well as clinical response. Also, dexamethasone lacks mineralocorticoid actively minimizing sodium and water retention. This may be clinically significant in treating patients with underlying cardiovascular disease or diseases associated with fluid retention (e.g. hypoalbuminemia or portal hypertension). The potency of dexamethasone is 4 to 10 times that of prednisone; therefore, a dose reduction is necessary when prescribing dexamethasone.[16,17]

In some patients, locally delivered GCs may be advantageous. Budesonide is an oral, locally active, high-potency GC that is formulated to exploit the pH differential between the proximal and distal small intestine, targeting budesonide's action to the distal intestinal tract. Budesonide is absorbed at the level of the enterocyte delivered by the portal system to the liver, where 80% to 90% of the absorbed budesonide undergoes first pass metabolism minimizing its systemic bioavailability. Some systemic absorption occurs, as evidence by a blunted ACTH (cosyntropin) stimulation test in dogs treated with budesonide at 3 mg/m^2 for 30 days.[18,19] Budesonide is used in management of Crohn disease in humans[20] and inflammatory bowel disease in dogs.[21] In dogs and cats with inflammatory respiratory disease, locally delivered fluticasone can be effectively inhaled to control clinical signs in patients with

Table 1
A comparison of potency, route of administration, site of action, and half-life of the more common glucocorticoids used in the treatment of immune-mediated or inflammatory diseases of dogs and cats

Type	Potency	Route of Administration	Site of Action	Biologic Half-life
Hydrocortisone/cortisol	1	IV	Systemic	8–12 h
Prednisone	4	PO	Systemic	12–36 h
Prednisolone	4	PO	Systemic	12–36 h
Dexamethasone	30	PO IV (SP)	Systemic	>48 h
Budesonide	60	PO	Intestinal Liver	$t_{1/2}$ = 2 h (canine)
Fluticasone	540	Inhaled	Lungs	$t_{1/2}$ = 8 h (human)

Abbreviation: dex SP = dexamethasone sodium phosphate.
Data from Kuchroo VK, Ohashi PS, Sartor RB, et al. Dysregulation of immune homeostasis in autoimmune diseases. Nat Med 2012;18(1):42–7.

GC-responsive inflammatory airway disease, which minimizes the adverse systemic side effects of GC therapy.[22–24]

Cyclosporine

Proposed mechanism

Cyclosporine is a polypeptide consisting of 11 amino acids, derived from a Norwegian soil fungus, *Tolypocladum inflatum*.[25] Cyclosporine inhibits the activation of T cells through the intracellular target calcineurin.[26,27] T lymphocytes express cyclophilin in high concentrations. Cyclophilin is an immunophilin or highly conserved protein that acts as a protein-folding enzyme (or proline isomerase).

Cyclosporine binds to cytoplasmic cyclophilin forming a cyclosporine-cyclophilin complex. The cyclosporine-cyclophilin complex binds and blocks the function of calcineurin, a serine/threonine phosphatase that is activated by increased intracellular calcium concentrations after T-cell receptor activation. Calcineurin functions to dephosphorylate the nuclear factor of activated T cells, enabling it to translocate into the nucleus, bind the nuclear transcription factor, activator protein 1, and induce transcription of genes for T-cell activation. The cyclosporine-cyclophilin complex prevents the dephosphorylation of nuclear factor of activated T cells, decreasing the expression of interleukin (IL)-2 and other cytokines, preventing further T-cell activation. Decreased IL-2 concentrations attenuate clonal proliferation of T lymphocytes and B lymphocytes. Cyclosporine also decreases the production of IL-3, IL-4, and tissue necrosis factor alpha, altering the function of granulocytes, macrophages, natural killer cells, eosinophils, and mast cells. In small animal veterinary species, cyclosporine is reported to decrease lymphocyte cytokine production in feline lymphocytes in vitro[28] and in canine lymphocytes in vitro and in vivo.[29,30]

Adverse effects/drug interactions

Historically, cyclosporine has been used for its GC-sparing effects, its rapid onset of immunosuppression, and the potential for less systemic adverse effects. Mild gastrointestinal upset after oral cyclosporine administration is the most common side effect reported in dogs and cats. It is often transient or responsive to dose reduction and does not require drug discontinuation. In some cases, more severe systemic side effects have been reported in cats and dogs, which require the discontinuation of cyclosporine to include gingival hyperplasia, opportunistic infections, hepatoxicity, and lymphoproliferative disorders.[31,32] Parenteral cyclosporine administration in a cat has been reported to cause anaphylaxis.[33] Another potential complication associated with cyclosporine administration in dogs is the potential for thromboembolic complications.[34] Similar thromboembolic complications have been reported in human transplant patients associated with cyclosporine administration.[35–37]

Cyclosporine is a substrate of cytochrome P450, family 3, subfamily A (CYP3A), and drug interactions associated with cyclosporine administration are reported due to either the inhibition or induction of the cytochrome P450 enzyme system. Cyclosporine is also a substrate of the drug transporter, P-glycoprotein, which also influences its disposition and leads to potential drug interactions. Clinically relevant drug interactions reported in dogs or cats as a result of the decreased cyclosporine metabolism and increased cyclosporine blood levels include its coadministration with azole antifungals,[38–41] clarithromycin,[42] and grapefruit juice.[43,44] The coadministration of cyclosporine with ketoconazole is often used therapeutically to decrease the dose and cost of cyclosporine while maintaining therapeutic blood levels.[40,41] The presumed mechanism of this exploited drug interaction is via inhibition of CYP3A and/or P-glycoprotein efflux.[45]

Clinical use

The initial use of cyclosporine in human and veterinary medicine was in the management of transplant recipients,[40,46] but more recently cyclosporine has been used in the treatment of inflammatory and immune-mediated diseases.

Specifically in veterinary medicine, cyclosporine is considered first-line therapy for perianal fistulas;[41,47-50] for keratoconjunctivitis sicca or dry eye;[51] and in some patients with atopic dermatitis.[52-54] The use of cyclosporine in the treatment of other inflammatory or immune-mediated diseases is as a second-line immunosuppressive agent based primarily on published retrospective case series. Examples include its use the treatment of feline and canine inflammatory bowel disease,[55] hemolytic anemia,[56] pure red cell aplasia,[33] and thrombocytopenia.[57]

Pharmacokinetics/pharmaceutics

The pharmacokinetics of cyclosporine is significantly impacted by the formulation (oil-based vs microemulsion), the species being treated, and the patient's intrinsic liver function/dysfunction or concurrently administered medications.[58] Despite the improvement in gastrointestinal absorption and intrapatient and interpatient variability in blood concentrations associated with the routine use of the microemulsion versus the oil-based formulation of cyclosporine, the disposition of cyclosporine remains variable. In some patients, therapeutic drug monitoring is indicated. Knowing a patient's history and concurrent medications, the cyclosporine formulation administered, and the assay method used for monitoring blood levels is essential. For example, the assays used to quantify cyclosporine blood levels vary depending on the compartment analyzed (plasma vs whole blood) and whether an immunoassay or a high-performance liquid chromatography method is used.[59]

In veterinary medicine, the targeted blood levels of cyclosporine necessary for the effective treatment of immune-mediated diseases are not as clearly established as they are in transplant medicine. A suggested therapeutic goal for cyclosporine in the treatment of immune-mediated cytopenias in humans is a whole-blood trough cyclosporine concentration between 150 ng/mL to 250 ng/mL for a maximum of 3 to 4 months followed by maintenance therapy with the minimum dosage to maintain remission.[60] No clinical therapeutic data are available for cyclosporine in the treatment of immune-mediated diseases in dogs and cats. Trough whole-blood cyclosporine levels between 400 ng/mL and 600 ng/mL are routinely used as the therapeutic target in veterinary medicine for efficacy and safety, which has been extrapolated from transplant patients.[29,61] Trough levels, however, often do not reliably predict clinical response. Research continues to explore immunosuppressive markers that parallel cyclosporine's clinical response, including the use of drug exposure,[62,63] T-cell cytokine expression,[29] and lymphocyte-specific proliferation.[64]

Tacrolimus is related to cyclosporine by its similar mechanism of action and immunosuppression. Tacrolimus also binds a cytoplasmic immunophilin, FKBP12, functioning as a potent immunosuppressive agent but has limited use in cats and dogs due to its severe systemic side effects. The clinical use of tacrolimus in veterinary medicine is as a topical therapy for perianal fistulas,[65] keratoconjunctivitis sicca,[66] or dermatitis.[53,67]

Azathioprine

Proposed mechanism

Azathioprine is a thiopurine that is a prodrug of 6-mercaptopurine.[68,69] In the liver and other peripheral tissues (e.g. erythrocytes), 6-mercaptopurine is enzymatically oxidized to inactive metabolites 6-thiouric acid via xanthine oxidase or methylated via thiopurine methyltransferase (TPMT) to 6-methylmercatopurine. The 6-thioguanine nucleotides (6-TGNs) are generated via hypoxanthine phosphoribosyl transferase, the active metabolites responsible for both the therapeutic and cytotoxic effects of azathioprine. 6-TGNs compete with endogenous purines for incorporation into RNA and DNA, creating nonfunctional DNA and RNA and disrupting DNA and RNA synthesis and mitosis. Azathioprine targets cell-mediated immunity, specifically lymphocytes, due to their lack of a salvage pathway for purine biosynthesis. Through its inhibition of de novo purine synthesis azathioprine interferes with lymphocyte proliferation, reduces lymphocyte numbers, and decreases T-cell–dependent antibody synthesis.

Adverse effects/drug interactions

The most common adverse effects attributed to azathioprine administration and subsequent drug withdrawal in humans and dogs include myelosuppression and gastrointestinal upset (vomiting and diarrhea).[70,71] Azathioprine myelosuppression is a delayed response, occurring after 1 to 2 weeks of therapy, which is reversible after drug withdrawal. One study reports a 13% prevalence of myelosuppression (dose-dependent neutropenia and thrombocytopenia) in dogs with immune-mediated hemolytic anemia (IMHA) treated with azathioprine and prednisone for 3 months.[72] Other less-common adverse effects include hepatic necrosis and pancreatitis.

Due to the risk of hepatitis and hepatic necrosis prior to and after the initiation of azathioprine therapy, monitoring liver enzymes is recommended. In humans, hepatotoxicity has been correlated with increased erythrocyte 6-methylmercaptopurine concentrations.[73] In rats, liver necrosis associated with azathioprine administration results in oxidative damage, glutathione depletion, and marked increases alanine aminotransaminase activity.[74]

Clinical use

In humans, azathioprine is used for the treatment of immune-mediated disease and organ transplant medicine.[75] Its use in treating immune-mediated diseases in dogs is in part due to its GC-sparing effect, which enables sustained disease remission while tapering or after GC withdrawal. Its effectiveness in the treatment of acute immune-mediated illness is limited based on its delayed efficacy of days to weeks.[76,77] Few controlled studies have been published evaluating the use of azathioprine in treating immune-mediated disease in dogs; therefore, its use is reliant on published retrospective studies reporting its use in the treatment of IMHA.[72,78,79]

Pharmacokinetics/pharmaceutics

In humans, TPMT activity is variable and correlates with clinical outcomes, including therapeutic efficacy and toxicity. Due to a genetic polymorphism, some individuals have increased or decreased TMPT activity. Decreased TMPT activity is associated with an increased risk of azathioprine-induced myelosuppression due to increased substrate availability for HRPT and the generation of cytotoxic 6-TGNs. A 9-fold difference in TPMT activity has been reported in dogs, with lower TMPT activity in giant schnauzers and higher TMPT activity in Alaskan malamutes.[80] Compared with dogs or humans, cats have decreased TMPT activity, which increases their risk of toxicity.[81,82] The use of azathioprine in cats is generally avoided and, if used, a significant dose reduction is recommended.

Allopurinol, a xanthine oxidase inhibitor, results in a significant increase in 6-TGN concentrations, increasing the risk of azathioprine toxicity (ie, myelosuppression). In humans, historically concurrent therapy of azathioprine with allopurinol was considered contraindicated or minimally required significant azathioprine dose reduction to avoid significant adverse drug-drug interactions.[83] In human patients with high TPMT activity and inflammatory bowel disease nonresponsive to azathioprine therapy, the concurrent administration of allopurinol with azathioprine has been exploited to increase the concentration of 6-TGNs and induce disease remission.[84–86]

Chlorambucil

Proposed mechanism
Chlorambucil is a nitrogen mustard derivative and prodrug that is converted in the liver to its active metabolite, phenylacetic acid. It is a cell-cycle nonspecific, cytotoxic, alkylating agent capable of cross-linking DNA. Chlorambucil targets B cells and is considered a slow-acting immunosuppressive agent that may require 2 weeks to reach therapeutic efficacy.

Adverse effects/drug interactions
Relative to azathioprine in cats, chlorambucil has less adverse side effects. Cytotoxic myelosuppression and gastrointestinal toxicity are associated with chlorambucil administration. Myelosuppression is considered mild and generally occurs 7 to 14 days after the start of therapy. Neurotoxicity (ie, reversible myoclonus) has been reported in a cat in association with a chlorambucil overdose.[87]

Clinical use
Prospective clinical studies evaluating the use of chlorambucil as an immunosuppressive agent are lacking. The majority of published studies in cats focus on the use of chlorambucil as a chemotherapeutic agent in the treatment of lymphoma.[88–90] Despite the paucity of data, chlorambucil is most often used as the cytotoxic drug of choice in cats. Its role as a second-line immunosuppressive therapy in cats has been used in the treatment of inflammatory bowel disease that is either severe or poorly responsive to prednisone/prednisolone therapy.[91–93] In a recent case series of cats with IMT, chlorambucil was successful as a second-tier drug in one cat that failed to achieve remission with prednisone alone.[94]

ADJUNCTIVE IMMUNOMODULATORY THERAPIES

In veterinary medicine, vincristine and human intravenous immunoglobulin (hIVIg) are considered adjunctive therapies to standard immunosuppressive protocols in the acute management of patients with immune-mediated diseases. Advantages include their potential for initial disease stabilization due to the potential for a relative fast therapeutic response as well as the low likelihood of adverse effects. Based on the limited objective published studies in veterinary medicine, the patient populations that may most likely benefit for either vincristine or IVIg are dogs with severe IMT. These include either dogs that failed to respond to standard immunosuppressive protocols or dogs in which their initial clinical presentation is severe, including a substantial risk of a fatal hemorrhage.[95,96] As in humans with immune thrombocytopenic purpura, these adjunctive agents are not typically useful as a single-agent therapy.[97]

Vincristine

Proposed mechanism
Vincristine is an alkaloid derived from the periwinkle plant. Several mechanisms have been proposed by which vincristine increases platelet counts, including stimulating megakaryocyte fragmentation and impairing microtubule assembly within macrophages, interfering with their ability to phagocytize optimized platelet. In humans, as

a single-agent therapy, vincristine only increases platelet counts in a subset of refractory patients with chronic thrombocytopenia.

Adverse effects/drug interactions
In dogs, the vincristine dose, 0.02 mg/kg, reported as used in the treatment of IMT, has not been associated with a clinically significant myelosuppression.[96] Other potential side effects of vincristine therapy include gastrointestinal upset (anorexia, vomiting, or diarrhea) or peripheral neuropathy (rare).[98,99] Extreme caution should be used during the administration of vincristine to avoid extravasation and perivascular sloughing.[100,101]

Clinical use
Vincristine's usefulness may be as emergent therapy in patients with IMT that are actively bleeding and transfusion dependent with evidence of megakaryocyte hyperplasia. Its use as an adjunctive therapy is to either initially increase platelet counts to enable initial patient stabilization while waiting for a clinical response from standard immune-mediated therapies or as a salvage therapy to increase platelet counts in patients with refractory immune mediated thrombocytopenia.[97,102,103]

In 24 dogs with severe IMT, Rozanski and colleagues[96] reported dogs treated with prednisone and vincristine experienced an increase in their platelet count to greater than 40,000/μL in a mean of 4.9 versus 6.8 days and a shorter duration of hospitalization a mean of 5.4 versus 7.3 days than dogs treated with prednisone alone. None of the dogs treated with vincristine experienced any adverse effects, including no increased risk of bleeding suggestive of altered platelet function after vincristine administration. The effect of vincristine on platelet function in dogs with IMT has not been evaluated. In healthy dogs, however, the administration of vincristine is reported to stimulate thrombopoiesis[102–105] and has no adverse affect in vivo platelet function.[105] This is in contrast to dogs with lymphoma in which the administration of vincristine results in abnormal platelet aggregation.[106]

Human Intravenous Immunoglobulin

Proposed mechanism
hIVIg is a purified product of pooled human plasma from multiple healthy donors. Approximately 90% of hIVIg is purified IgG with trace concentrations of IgA, IgM, CD4, CD8, and HLA molecules.[107] In the treatment of immune-mediated diseases, hIVIg is used for its ability to regulate the immune system, inhibit phagocytosis, and decrease tissue damage.[108–110] The immunomodulatory actions of hIVIg are not well understood but the efficacy of hIVIg therapy in the treatment of immune-mediated diseases has been attributed to multiple mechanisms. Some of the dominant mechanisms of action of hIVIg include Fc receptor blockade, autoantibody elimination, cytokine modulation, complement inhibition, and Fas–Fas ligand blockade.

Adverse effects/drug interactions
The most anticipated adverse effect of hIVIg in veterinary patients is the risk of an acute hypersensitivity reaction due to the infusion of human-derived foreign proteins into canine or feline species. Other adverse effects reported in human patients treated with hIVIg include hypotension,[111] thromboembolism,[112] renal insufficiency,[113] and dose-dependent aseptic meningitis.[114] In human patients, a decrease in acute hypersensitivity reactions and other adverse effects are associated with the use of hIVIg products that have been processed to remove the IgG aggregates or contain low IVIg concentrations and with the use of non–sucrose-containing products as well as the use of slow infusion rates.[109,115]

No significant adverse effects have been reported in association with hIVIG administration in clinically ill dogs and cats.[95,116–120] Of the reported studies available, however, different doses and hIVIg products were used and, in some of the canine studies, diphenhydramine was administered prior to the infusion of hIVIg,[95,121,122] making the true assessment of the adverse effects of hIVIg difficult. An experimental study in healthy beagles supports an inflammatory/hypercoagulable state after the administration of hIVIg.[123] Conclusive clinical studies in dogs, specifically in dogs with concurrent prothrombotic conditions, are lacking.[124] In addition, limited data are available on the safety of repeated or multiple hIVIg transfusion in dogs.[116–118,120,125] and more studies are necessary to assess the risk before repeated hIVIg infusions can be recommended.

Clinical use

The use of hIVIg in humans initially began in the treatment of immunodeficiency disorders but now includes a wide range of immune-mediated and inflammatory disorders despite the limited number of Food and Drug Administration–approved conditions.[126–130] The 7 approved conditions for hIVIg use in human patients included Kawasaki disease, bone marrow transplantation, idiopathic thrombocytopenic purpura, chronic B-cell lymphocytic leukemia, pediatric HIV, chronic inflammatory demyelinating polyneuropathy, and primary immunoglobulin deficiency.[128]

Canine lymphocytes and monocytes have been shown to be effectively bound by.[131] The first reports of the clinical use of hIVIg in veterinary medicine were in dogs with immune-mediated hemolytic anemia.[119,132] The use of hIVIg in veterinary medicine has since expanded to its use as an adjunctive therapy in a variety of immune-mediated diseases, including hemolytic anemia,[56,124] thrombocytopenia,[95,121] immune-mediated cutaneous diseases,[116,118,120,125] and sudden acquired retinal degeneration syndrome.[117]

The potential advantage of hIVIg is the ability of IgG to quickly block the Fc receptor and provide initial disease stabilization by decreasing immune-mediated destruction and continued tissue injury. This initial patient stabilization provides time for the traditional long-term immuomodulatory therapies to become clinically effective, shortens hospitalization, and decreases the dependence on repeated transfusions and additional supportive care.[116,118–121,125] No consensus on the use of hIVIg in veterinary patients with immune-mediated diseases has been established because most data are limited to retrospective studies,[119,121,133] case reports,[95,116,118,125] and few prospective, randomized, investigator-blinded, placebo-controlled clinical trials.[122,124]

A prospective, randomized, double-blinded, placebo controlled clinical trial has been published supporting the use of hIVIg in dogs with IMT. Bianco and colleagues[122] treated all dogs with severe IMT with immunosuppressive doses of prednisone, then randomized the dogs to either placebo or a single infusion of hIVIg within 24 hours of the initiation of prednisone therapy. The dogs treated with prednisone and hIVIG had a significant reduction in time to resolution of their thrombocytopenia (mean 3.7 vs 7.5 days; $P = .0180$) and number of days hospitalized (mean 4 vs 8 days; $P = .0270$) compared with dogs treated with prednisone alone. There was no significant difference, however, in the number of blood transfusions, cost, or mortality. Treatment of dogs with severe IMT with prednisone and hIVIg resulted in similar response times and days of hospitalization as reported for canine patients with IMT treated with prednisone and vincristine by Rozanski and colleagues[96] (**Table 2**). Further studies are needed to identify if hIVIg has benefits over vincristine in treating dogs with severe IMT.

Table 2
Initial stabilization of canine immune-mediated thrombocytopenia, a comparison of days to platelet recovery and duration of hospitalization for dogs treated with prednisone in addition to adjunctive therapies, vincristine versus human intravenous immunoglobulin (hIVIg)

Study	Prednisone (3 mg/kg/d)		(+) Vincristine (0.02 mg/kg IV)		(+) hIVIG (0.5 g/kg IV)	
	>40 K/uL plt (days)	ICU (days)	>40 K/uL plt (days)	ICU (days)	>40 K/uL plt (days)	ICU (days)
Rozanski et al,[96] 2002 (n = 24)	6.8 ± 4.5	7.3 ± 0.5	4.9 ± 1.1	5.4 ± 0.3	—	—
Bianco et al,[122] 2009 (n = 18)	7.8 ± 3.9	8.3 ± 0.6	—	—	3.7 ± 1.3	4.2 ± 0.4

Abbreviation: plt = platelets.
Data reported as mean ± SD.

In a blinded clinical trial, 28 dogs with IMHA were randomized to either treatment with hIVIg versus placebo (0.9% NaCl) as part of their initial drug therapy and disease stabilization.[124] All dogs were treated concurrently with prednisone and low-molecular-weight heparin. There was no difference in days to stabilization of PCV or duration of hospitalization between the 2 treatment groups.

Pharmacokinetics/pharmaceutics
A range of hIVIg products is available with varying IgG concentrations, osmolality, and sugar content.[134] The dose and duration of hIVIg infusions in veterinary patients have been extrapolated from its use in human medicine. Published reports in dogs and cats have used doses ranging from 0.25 g/kg to 2.2 g/kg, with infusion durations ranging from 4 hours to 12 hours.[116–120,122] The specific hIVIg products used have varied as well. The use of hIVIg products in clinical veterinary medicine may be more a function of its availability to veterinary clinicians and the dose used may be influenced by cost. In many cases, the use of hIVIg may be cost prohibitive in veterinary patients.

EMERGING IMMUNOSUPPRESSIVE THERAPIES
Mycophenolate Mofetil

Proposed mechanism
Mycophenolate mofetil (MMF), the prodrug of mycophenolic acid (MPA), is used in human medicine as an alternative immunosuppressant to azathioprine in transplant medicine[135–137] and in the treatment of immune-mediated diseases.[138–140] MPA is a potent, selective, noncompetitive, reversible inhibitor of inosine-5′-monophosphate dehydrogenase (IMPDH), specifically, the type II isoform of IMPDH.[26,140] The IMPDH type II isoform is more abundant in activated lymphocytes and is 5 times more susceptible to MPA than the type I isoform (expressed in many cell types). IMPDH catalyzes the rate-limiting step of the de novo biosynthesis of guanosine nucleotides, which converts inosine monophosphate to guanosine monophosphate. MPA's cytotoxicity is selective to lymphocytes via the depletion of guanosine and deoxyguanosine nucleotides. T lymphocytes and B lymphocytes are entirely dependent on the de novo pathway for purine synthesis, differentiation, proliferation, and immunoglobulin production. Other mechanisms that contribute to MMF's effectiveness in treating inflammatory and immune-mediated diseases are via its suppression of dendritic cell maturation and reduction in monocyte recruitment into the site of inflammation.[141]

In addition, MMF may be antifibrotic through its ability to inhibit proliferation of non–immune cells, including smooth muscle, renal tubular, and mesangial cells.[142]

Adverse effects/drug interactions

Side effects reported in humans treated with MMF include gastrointestinal upset, opportunistic infections, allergic reactions, neutropenia, and lymphoma.[140,143] Limited information is available about the adverse effects of MMF in dogs and cats. The primary side effects reported in dogs treated with oral MMF are diarrhea and weight loss.[144,145] Mild allergic reactions have been reported with the administration of parenteral MMF in dogs.[146]

Drug interactions reported in humans treated with MMF resulting in decreased MMF's bioavailability may also be clinically relevant in veterinary patients. The concurrent administration with some antibiotics (ie, fluoroquinolones and metronidazole) reduces the enterohepatic circulation of MMF.[147] If an enteric-coated formulation of oral MMF is not used, the higher gastric pH achieved with proton pump inhibitors reduces the dissolution of MMF and decreases drug exposure.[148] Cyclosporine decreases MMF exposure via inhibition of the enterohepatic recirculation of MMF due to reduced biliary excretion of the glucuronide metabolite by multidrug resistance protein 2 transporter.[149] GCs induce the uridine diphosphate glucuronosyltransferase enzyme system, increasing the metabolism of MMF.[150] Consideration should be given to possible drug-drug interactions in patients nonresponsive to MMF. The concurrent use of MMF with azathioprine is not recommended based on their similar mechanism of action and risk of bone marrow suppression.[140]

Clinical use

The use of mycophenolate in dogs and cats with refractory inflammatory or immune-mediated diseases continue to emerge in the literature as case reports or case series. Canine diseases reported as responsive to MMF include aplastic anemia[151] and subepidermal blistering autoimmune skin disease.[152] Recently, a case report was published describing the successful use of MMF in 2 cats with refractory immune-mediated hemolytic anemia.[153] A small retrospective case series evaluating dogs with acquired myasthenia gravis treated with mycophenolate and pyridostigmine versus pyridostigmine alone was not supportive of the use of MMF based on no differences in remission rates, time to remission, and survival.[145]

Pharmacokinetics/pharmaceutics

In veterinary patients MMF is anticipated to have a rapid onset of action (maximal IMPDH inhibition 2–4 hours post oral administration) and acceptable tolerability.[146,154,155]

Leflunomide

Proposed mechanism

Leflunomide is a synthetic isoxazole derivative that is metabolized to its active metabolite, malononitrilamide, or teriflunomide.[156–158] Teriflunomide primarily functions as a selective pyrimidine synthesis inhibitor via the reversible inhibition of dihydroorotate dehydrogenase, a mitochondrial enzyme required for de novo pyrimidine biosynthesis. Other possible mechanisms of actions include inhibition of tyrosine kinase activity, which alters cytokine and growth factor receptors associated with tyrosine kinase activity. Leflunomide targets B lymphocytes and T lymphocytes, which lack a pyrimidine salvage pathway. In vitro canine B and T cells were sensitive to the antiproliferative effects of malononitrilamide.[159] In a dose-dependent manner, malononitrilamide has been reported to inhibit mitogen-stimulated proliferation of feline lymphocytes in vitro.[160]

Adverse effects/drug interactions

Reported clinical side effects in dogs include lethargy, gastrointestinal upset, and mild bone marrow suppression (leukopenia and thrombocytopenia).[161,162] Dose-dependent myelosuppression has been reported in dogs treated with leflunomide at dosages greater than or equal to 4 mg/kg once a day.[163] Anecdotal reports of severe myelosuppression (ie, leukopenia) and in some cases bone marrow necrosis have been associated with leflunomide therapy in dogs. In humans, severe idiosyncratic reactions have been reported with leflunomide therapy, including myelosuppression, hepatotoxicosis, and toxic epidermal necrolysis.[156,157]

Clinical use

Leflunomide has been used in humans for its immunosuppressive and antiproliferative effects in the treatment of rheumatoid arthritis, Crohn disease, and systemic lupus erythematosus and the management of transplant receipients.[156,157] Gregory and colleagues[162] initially described the use of use leflunomide as an add-on therapy for a variety of naturally occurring immune mediated/inflammatory disease in dogs, including IMT, immune-mediated hemolytic anemia, systemic histiocytosis, nonsuppurative encephalitis/meningomyelitis, immune-mediated polymyositis, immune-mediated polyarthritis, and pemphigus foliaceus. Additional case reports and retrospective studies have been published describing the successful use of leflunomide in companion animal medicine. Leflunomide has been used in the treatment of reactive histiocytosis,[164] and Evans syndrome[95] in dogs. A retrospective clinical study evaluating leflunomide in the treatment of immune-mediated polyarthritis was recently published;[161] 8 of the 14 dogs with immune-mediated polyarthritis had resolution of their clinical signs after the introduction of leflunomide. In a group of cats (n = 12) with rheumatoid arthritis, previously nonresponsive to standard therapy, leflunomide was used in conjunction with methotrexate to provide marked clinical improvement in half the cats.[165]

SUMMARY

The treatment of immune-mediated disease in dogs and cats continues to evolve as new therapies are introduced or adapted from human medicine. GCs remain the first-line therapy for many of the immune-mediated or inflammatory diseases of cats and dogs. Therapies incorporating cyclosporine, azathioprine, or chlorambucil are the more common second-line therapies used, but their use is clinician and patient dependent. Often, these second-line therapies are introduced due to a patient's lack of response or intolerable side effects associated with GC therapy or may be introduced early in the disease process due to a patient's severe life-threatening clinical presentation. **Table 3** summarizes and compares the more common non-GC immunosuppressive drugs used in dogs and cats. The introduction of adjunctive therapies (vincristine and hIVIG) aid in the initial disease stabilization and may decrease the duration of hospitalization and need for prolonged intensive supportive care. In dogs, the benefits of adjunctive therapies are best documented for idiopathic IMT.

For those refractory patients or patients with intolerable side effects associated with the standard immunosuppressive therapies, veterinary medicine continues to borrow alternative immunosuppressive agents from the experience of human medicine as new drugs continue to emerge. As emerging immunosuppressive therapeutics for veterinary patients are initially adopted, knowledge of their therapeutic efficacy and

Table 3
A comparison of mechanism of action, reported dosages, reported indications, adverse effects, and possible drug-drug interactions for the more common nonglucocorticoid immunosuppressive therapies used in the treatment of immune-mediated or inflammatory disease of dogs and cats

Drug	MOA	Dosage(s)	Indications	Adverse Effects
Cyclosporine	Calcineurin inhibitor	2.5 mg/kg PO q 12 h (with ketoconazole) or 4 mg/kg PO q 12 h 5 mg/kg PO q 24 h 5 mg/kg PO q 12 h 4 mg/kg PO q 12 h	Canine—perianal fistulas[41,48] Canine—IBD[55] Canine—IMHA[56] Feline—PRCA[33]	GI upset, gingival hyperplasia, hepatotoxicity, opportunistic infections, anaphylaxis (IV) Potential drug interactions—ketoconazole, clarithromycin, grapefruit juice
Azathioprine	Thiopurine analog—disrupts DNA/RNA synthesis	2 mg/kg PO q 24 h × 7–14 days then 2 mg/kg PO EOD	Canine—IMHA[72]	GI upset, myelosuppression, hepatic necrosis Potential drug interactions—allopurinol
Chlorambucil	Alkylating agent—cell-cycle nonspecific	0.02 mg/kg PO q 24 h × 7 d then 0.01 mg/kg 2 mg/cat PO q 48–72 h × 7–14 days then 2 mg/kg PO EOD or 20 mg/m² PO q 14 d	Feline—IMT[94] Feline—IBD[92]	GI upset, myelosuppression
MMF	Purine synthesis inhibitor	10 mg/kg PO q 12 h 10 mg/kg PO q 12 h	Canine—aplastic anemia[151] Feline—IMHA[153]	Allergic reaction, diarrhea, weight loss Potential drug interactions—FQ, metronidazole, PPIs, GC, cyclosporine
Leflunomide	Pyrimidine synthesis inhibitor	2–4 mg/kg PO q 24 h 10 mg/cat PO q 24 h	Canine—IMPA[161] Feline—RA[165]	Lethargy, GI upset, myelosuppression

Abbreviations: FQ, fluoroquinolone; GI, gastrointestinal; IBD, inflammatory bowel disease; IMPA, immune mediated polyarthritis; MOA, mechanism of action; PPIs, proton pump inhibitors; PRCA, pure red cell aplasia; RA, rheumatoid arthritis.

potential for adverse effects remains limited. Ultimately, the goals of any immunosuppressive treatment protocol are to initially achieve disease remission while minimizing adverse effects, followed by a gradual taper of drugs to the lowest doses to maintain disease remission or, in some cases, successful drug withdrawal.

REFERENCES

1. Kuchroo VK, Ohashi PS, Sartor RB, et al. Dysregulation of immune homeostasis in autoimmune diseases. Nat Med 2012;18(1):42–7.
2. Davidson A, Diamond B. Autoimmune diseases. N Engl J Med 2001;345(5): 340–50.
3. Gershwin LJ. Autoimmune diseases in small animals. Vet Clin North Am Small Anim Pract 2010;40(3):439–57.
4. Ferguson D, Dirikolu L, Hoenig M. Glucocorticoids, mineralocorticoids, adrenolytic drugs. In: Riviere JE, Papich MG, editors. Veterinary pharmacology and therapeutics. 9th edition. Ames (IO): Wiley-Blackwll; 2009. p. 771–802.
5. Zen M, Canova M, Campana C, et al. The kaleidoscope of glucorticoid effects on immune system. Autoimmun Rev 2011;10(6):305–10.
6. Ashwell JD, Lu FW, Vacchio MS. Glucocorticoids in T cell development and function*. Annu Rev Immunol 2000;18:309–45.
7. Al-Ghazlat S. Immunosuppressive therapy for canine immune-mediated hemolytic anemia. Compend Contin Educ Vet 2009;31(1):33–41.
8. Buttgereit F, Scheffold A. Rapid glucocorticoid effects on immune cells. Steroids 2002;67(6):529–34.
9. Friedman D, Netti F, Schreiber AD. Effect of estradiol and steroid analogues on the clearance of immunoglobulin G-coated erythrocytes. J Clin Invest 1985; 75(1):162–7.
10. Gernsheimer T, Stratton J, Ballem PJ, et al. Mechanisms of response to treatment in autoimmune thrombocytopenic purpura. N Engl J Med 1989;320(15): 974–80.
11. Miller E. Immunosuppressive therapy in the treatment of immune-mediated disease. J Vet Intern Med 1992;6(4):206–13.
12. Galon J, Franchimont D, Hiroi N, et al. Gene profiling reveals unknown enhancing and suppressive actions of glucocorticoids on immune cells. FASEB J 2002;16(1):61–71.
13. Boston SE, Moens NM, Kruth SA, et al. Endoscopic evaluation of the gastroduodenal mucosa to determine the safety of short-term concurrent administration of meloxicam and dexamethasone in healthy dogs. Am J Vet Res 2003;64(11): 1369–75.
14. Plumb DC. Plumb's veterinary drug Handbook. Ames (IA): Iowa State University Press; 2011.
15. Graham-Mize C, Rosser E. Bioavailability and activity of prednisone and prednisolone in the feline patient [abstract]. Vet Dermatol 2004;15:7.
16. Ballard PL, Carter JP, Graham BS, et al. A radioreceptor assay for evaluation of the plasma glucocorticoid activity of natural and synthetic steroids in man. J Clin Endocrinol Metab 1975;41(2):290–304.
17. Cantrill HL, Waltman SR, Palmberg PF, et al. In vitro determination of relative corticosteroid potency. J Clin Endocrinol Metab 1975;40(6):1073–7.
18. Stroup ST, Behrend EN, Kemppainen RJ, et al. Effects of oral administration of controlled-ileal-release budesonide and assessment of pituitary-adrenocortical axis suppression in clinically normal dogs. Am J Vet Res 2006;67(7):1173–8.

19. Tumulty JW, Broussard JD, Steiner JM, et al. Clinical effects of short-term oral budesonide on the hypothalamic-pituitary-adrenal axis in dogs with inflammatory bowel disease. J Am Anim Hosp Assoc 2004;40(2):120–3.

20. De Cassan C, Fiorino G, Danese S. Second-generation corticosteroids for the treatment of Crohn's disease and ulcerative colitis: more effective and less side effects? Dig Dis 2012;30(4):368–75.

21. Pietra M, Fracassi F, Diana A, et al. Plasma concentrations and therapeutic effects of budesonide in dogs with inflammatory bowel disease. Am J Vet Res 2013;74(1):78–83.

22. Bexfield NH, Foale RD, Davison LJ, et al. Management of 13 cases of canine respiratory disease using inhaled corticosteroids. J Small Anim Pract 2006; 47(7):377–82.

23. Cohn LA, DeClue AE, Cohen RL, et al. Effects of fluticasone propionate dosage in an experimental model of feline asthma. J Feline Med Surg 2010; 12(2):91–6.

24. Leemans J, Kirschvink N, Clercx C, et al. Effect of short-term oral and inhaled corticosteroids on airway inflammation and responsiveness in a feline acute asthma model. Vet J 2012;192(1):41–8.

25. Stahelin H. Cyclosporin A. Historical background. Prog Allergy 1986;38:19–27.

26. Halloran PF. Molecular mechanisms of new immunosuppressants. Clin Transplant 1996;10:118–23.

27. Whitley NT, Day MJ. Immunomodulatory drugs and their application to the management of canine immune-mediated disease. J Small Anim Pract 2011;52(2): 70–85.

28. Aronson LR, Stumhofer JS, Drobatz KJ, et al. Effect of cyclosporine, dexamethasone, and human CTLA4-Ig on production of cytokines in lymphocytes of clinically normal cats and cats undergoing renal transplantation. Am J Vet Res 2011;72(4):541–9.

29. Archer TM, Fellman CL, Stokes JV, et al. Pharmacodynamic monitoring of canine T-cell cytokine responses to oral cyclosporine. J Vet Intern Med 2011;25(6): 1391–7.

30. Fellman CL, Stokes JV, Archer TM, et al. Cyclosporine A affects the in vitro expression of T cell activation-related molecules and cytokines in dogs. Vet Immunol Immunopathol 2011;140(3–4):175–80.

31. Robson D. Review of the pharmacokinetics, interactions and adverse reactions of cyclosporine in people, dogs and cats. Vet Rec 2003;152(24):739–48.

32. Schmiedt CW, Grimes JA, Holzman G, et al. Incidence and risk factors for development of malignant neoplasia after feline renal transplantation and cyclosporine-based immunosuppression. Vet Comp Oncol 2009;7(1):45–53.

33. Viviano KR, Webb JL. Clinical use of cyclosporine as an adjunctive therapy in the management of feline idiopathic pure red cell aplasia. J Feline Med Surg 2011;13(12):885–95.

34. Thomason J, Lunsford K, Stokes J, et al. The effects of cyclosporine on platelet function and cyclooxygenase expression in normal dogs. J Vet Intern Med 2012; 26(6):1389–401.

35. Averna M, Barbagallo CM, Ganci A, et al. Determinants of enhanced thromboxane biosynthesis in renal transplantation. Kidney Int 2001;59(4): 1574–9.

36. Jespersen B, Thiesson HC, Henriksen C, et al. Differential effects of immunosuppressive drugs on COX-2 activity in vitro and in kidney transplant patients in vivo. Nephrol Dial Transplant 2009;24(5):1644–55.

37. Sahin G, Akay OM, Kus E, et al. Effects of immunosuppressive drugs on platelet aggregation and soluble P-selectin levels in renal transplant patients. Ren Fail 2009;31(2):111–7.

38. Katayama M, Igarashi H, Fukai K, et al. Fluconazole decreases cyclosporine dosage in renal transplanted dogs. Res Vet Sci 2010;89(1):124–5.

39. Katayama M, Katayama R, Kamishina H. Effects of multiple oral dosing of itraconazole on the pharmacokinetics of cyclosporine in cats. J Feline Med Surg 2010;12(6):512–4.

40. McAnulty JF, Lensmeyer GL. The effects of ketoconazole on the pharmacokinetics of cyclosporine A in cats. Vet Surg 1999;28(6):448–55.

41. Patricelli AJ, Hardie RJ, McAnulty JE. Cyclosporine and ketoconazole for the treatment of perianal fistulas in dogs. J Am Vet Med Assoc 2002;220(7):1009–16.

42. Katayama M, Nishijima N, Okamura Y, et al. Interaction of clarithromycin with cyclosporine in cats: pharmacokinetic study and case report. J Feline Med Surg 2012;14(4):257–61.

43. Amatori FM, Meucci V, Giusiani M, et al. Effect of grapefruit juice on the pharmacokinetics of cyclosporine in dogs. Vet Rec 2004;154(6):180–1.

44. Radwanski NE, Cerundolo R, Shofer FS, et al. Effects of powdered whole grapefruit and metoclopramide on the pharmacokinetics of cyclosporine in dogs. Am J Vet Res 2011;72(5):687–93.

45. Trepanier LA. Cytochrome P450 and its role in veterinary drug interactions. Vet Clin North Am Small Anim Pract 2006;36(5):975–85, v.

46. Calne RY, White DJ, Thiru S, et al. Cyclosporin A in patients receiving renal allografts from cadaver donors. Lancet 1978;2(8104–5):1323–7.

47. Griffiths LG, Sullivan M, Borland WW. Cyclosporin as the sole treatment for anal furunculosis: preliminary results. J Small Anim Pract 1999;40(12):569–72.

48. Hardie RJ, Gregory SP, Tomlin J, et al. Cyclosporine treatment of anal furunculosis in 26 dogs. J Small Anim Pract 2005;46(1):3–9.

49. Mathews KA, Sukhiani HR. Randomized controlled trial of cyclosporine for treatment of perianal fistulas in dogs. J Am Vet Med Assoc 1997;211(10):1249–53.

50. O'Neill T, Edwards GA, Holloway S. Efficacy of combined cyclosporine A and ketoconazole treatment of anal furunculosis. J Small Anim Pract 2004;45(5):238–43.

51. Moore CP. Immunomodulating agents. Vet Clin North Am Small Anim Pract 2004;34(3):725–37.

52. Guaguere E, Steffan J, Olivry T. Cyclosporin A: a new drug in the field of canine dermatology. Vet Dermatol 2004;15(2):61–74.

53. Olivry T, Foster AP, Mueller RS, et al. Interventions for atopic dermatitis in dogs: a systematic review of randomized controlled trials. Vet Dermatol 2010;21(1):4–22.

54. Steffan J, Favrot C, Mueller R. A systemic review and meta-analysis of the efficacy and safety of cyclosporin for the treatment of atopic dermatitis in dogs. Vet Dermatol 2006;17:3–16.

55. Allenspach K, Rufenacht S, Sauter S, et al. Pharmacokinetics and clinical efficacy of cyclosporine treatment of dogs with steroid-refractory inflammatory bowel disease. J Vet Intern Med 2006;20(2):239–44.

56. Grundy SA, Barton C. Influence of drug treatment on survival of dogs with immune-mediated hemolytic anemia: 88 cases (1989-1999). J Am Vet Med Assoc 2001;218(4):543–6.

57. Nakamura RK, Tompkins E, Bianco D. Therapeutic options for immune-mediated thrombocytopenia. J Vet Emerg Crit Care (San Antonio) 2012;22(1):59–72.

58. Whalen RD, Tata PN, Burckart GJ, et al. Species differences in the hepatic and intestinal metabolism of cyclosporine. Xenobiotica 1999;29(1):3–9.
59. Trifilio SM, Scheetz M, Borensztajn J, et al. Variability of cyclosporine concentrations by HPLC and TDX monoclonal assay methods, application of a correction factor, and description of a novel clinical approach to determine the practical consequences of changing assay technique. Clin Transplant 2013;27(1):154–61.
60. Teramura M, Kimura A, Iwase S, et al. Treatment of severe aplastic anemia with antithymocyte globulin and cyclosporin A with or without G-CSF in adults: a multicenter randomized study in Japan. Blood 2007;110(6):1756–61.
61. Nam HS, McAnulty JF, Kwak HH, et al. Gingival overgrowth in dogs associated with clinically relevant cyclosporine blood levels: observations in a canine renal transplantation model. Vet Surg 2008;37(3):247–53.
62. Mehl ML, Kyles AE, Craigmill AL, et al. Disposition of cyclosporine after intravenous and multi-dose oral administration in cats. J Vet Pharmacol Ther 2003; 26(5):349–54.
63. Nashan B, Cole E, Levy G, et al. Clinical validation studies of Neoral C(2) monitoring: a review. Transplantation 2002;73(Suppl 9):S3–11.
64. Nafe LA, Dodam JR, Reinero CR. Ex Vivo immunosuppression of canine T lymphocyte-specific proliferation using dexamethasone, cyclosporine, and active metabolites of azathioprine and leflunomide in a flow cytometric assay. Paper presented at: 2012 Proceedings ACVIM. New Orleans, LA. ACVIM Forum, May 30-June 2, 2012.
65. Stanley BJ, Hauptman JG. Long-term prospective evaluation of topically applied 0.1% tacrolimus ointment for treatment of perianal sinuses in dogs. J Am Vet Med Assoc 2009;235(4):397–404.
66. Hendrix DV, Adkins EA, Ward DA, et al. An investigation comparing the efficacy of topical ocular application of tacrolimus and cyclosporine in dogs. Vet Med Int 2011;2011:487592.
67. Chung TH, Ryu MH, Kim DY, et al. Topical tacrolimus (FK506) for the treatment of feline idiopathic facial dermatitis. Aust Vet J 2009;87(10):417–20.
68. Aarbakke J, Janka-Schaub G, Elion GB. Thiopurine biology and pharmacology. Trends Pharmacol Sci 1997;18(1):3–7.
69. Elion GB. The George Hitchings and Gertrude Elion Lecture. The pharmacology of azathioprine. Ann N Y Acad Sci 1993;685:400–7.
70. Houston DM, Taylor JA. Acute pancreatitis and bone marrow suppression in a dog given azathioprine. Can Vet J 1991;32(8):496–7.
71. Schwab M, Schaffeler E, Marx C, et al. Azathioprine therapy and adverse drug reactions in patients with inflammatory bowel disease: impact of thiopurine S-methyltransferase polymorphism. Pharmacogenetics 2002;12(6): 429–36.
72. Piek CJ, Junius G, Dekker A, et al. Idiopathic immune-mediated hemolytic anemia: treatment outcome and prognostic factors in 149 dogs. J Vet Intern Med 2008;22(2):366–73.
73. Dubinsky MC, Lamothe S, Yang HY, et al. Pharmacogenomics and metabolite measurement for 6-mercaptopurine therapy in inflammatory bowel disease. Gastroenterology 2000;118(4):705–13.
74. El-Beshbishy HA, Tork OM, El-Bab MF, et al. Antioxidant and antiapoptotic effects of green tea polyphenols against azathioprine-induced liver injury in rats. Pathophysiology 2011;18(2):125–35.
75. Kruh J, Foster CS. Corticosteroid-sparing agents: conventional systemic immunosuppressants. Dev Ophthalmol 2012;51:29–46.

76. Harkin KR, Phillips D, Wilkerson M. Evaluation of azathioprine on lesion severity and lymphocyte blastogenesis in dogs with perianal fistulas. J Am Anim Hosp Assoc 2007;43(1):21–6.
77. Ogilvie GK, Felsburg PJ, Harris CW. Short-term effect of cyclophosphamide and azathioprine on selected aspects of the canine blastogenic response. Vet Immunol Immunopathol 1988;18(2):119–27.
78. Reimer ME, Troy GC, Warnick LD. Immune-mediated hemolytic anemia: 70 cases (1988-1996). J Am Anim Hosp Assoc 1999;35(5):384–91.
79. Weinkle TK, Center SA, Randolph JF, et al. Evaluation of prognostic factors, survival rates, and treatment protocols for immune-mediated hemolytic anemia in dogs: 151 cases (1993-2002). J Am Vet Med Assoc 2005;226(11):1869–80.
80. Kidd LB, Salavaggione OE, Szumlanski CL, et al. Thiopurine methyltransferase activity in red blood cells of dogs. J Vet Intern Med 2004;18(2):214–8.
81. Beale KM, Altman D, Clemmons RR, et al. Systemic toxicosis associated with azathioprine administration in domestic cats. Am J Vet Res 1992;53(7): 1236–40.
82. Salavaggione OE, Yang C, Kidd LB, et al. Cat red blood cell thiopurine S-methyltransferase: companion animal pharmacogenetics. J Pharmacol Exp Ther 2004;308(2):617–26.
83. Berns A, Rubenfeld S, Rymzo WT Jr, et al. Hazard of combining allopurinol and thiopurine. N Engl J Med 1972;286(13):730–1.
84. Ansari A, Elliott T, Baburajan B, et al. Long-term outcome of using allopurinol cotherapy as a strategy for overcoming thiopurine hepatotoxicity in treating inflammatory bowel disease. Aliment Pharmacol Ther 2008;28(6):734–41.
85. Govani SM, Higgins PD. Combination of thiopurines and allopurinol: adverse events and clinical benefit in IBD. J Crohns Colitis 2010;4(4):444–9.
86. Sparrow MP, Hande SA, Friedman S, et al. Allopurinol safely and effectively optimizes tioguanine metabolites in inflammatory bowel disease patients not responding to azathioprine and mercaptopurine. Aliment Pharmacol Ther 2005; 22(5):441–6.
87. Benitah N, de Lorimier LP, Gaspar M, et al. Chlorambucil-induced myoclonus in a cat with lymphoma. J Am Anim Hosp Assoc 2003;39(3):283–7.
88. Barrs VR, Beatty JA. Feline alimentary lymphoma: 2. Further diagnostics, therapy and prognosis. J Feline Med Surg 2012;14(3):191–201.
89. Kiselow MA, Rassnick KM, McDonough SP, et al. Outcome of cats with low-grade lymphocytic lymphoma: 41 cases (1995-2005). J Am Vet Med Assoc 2008;232(3):405–10.
90. Lingard AE, Briscoe K, Beatty JA, et al. Low-grade alimentary lymphoma: clinicopathological findings and response to treatment in 17 cases. J Feline Med Surg 2009;11(8):692–700.
91. Jergens AE. Feline idiopathic inflammatory bowel disease: what we know and what remains to be unraveled. J Feline Med Surg 2012;14(7):445–58.
92. Trepanier L. Idiopathic inflammatory bowel disease in cats. Rational treatment selection. J Feline Med Surg 2009;11(1):32–8.
93. Willard MD. Feline inflammatory bowel disease: a review. J Feline Med Surg 1999;1(3):155–64.
94. Wondratschek C, Weingart C, Kohn B. Primary immune-mediated thrombocytopenia in cats. J Am Anim Hosp Assoc 2010;46(1):12–9.
95. Bianco D, Hardy RM. Treatment of Evans' syndrome with human intravenous immunoglobulin and leflunomide in a diabetic dog. J Am Anim Hosp Assoc 2009;45(3):147–50.

96. Rozanski EA, Callan MB, Hughes D, et al. Comparison of platelet count recovery with use of vincristine and prednisone or prednisone alone for treatment for severe immune-mediated thrombocytopenia in dogs. J Am Vet Med Assoc 2002; 220(4):477–81.

97. Boruchov DM, Gururangan S, Driscoll MC, et al. Multiagent induction and maintenance therapy for patients with refractory immune thrombocytopenic purpura (ITP). Blood 2007;110(10):3526–31.

98. Golden DL, Langston VC. The use of vincristine and vinblastine in dogs and cats. J Am Vet Med Assoc 1988;93:1114–7.

99. Wohl JS, Cotter SM. Approach to complications of anticancer therapy in emergency practice. J Vet Emerg Crit Care 1995;5:61–76.

100. Schulmeister L. Extravasation management: clinical update. Semin Oncol Nurs 2011;27(1):82–90.

101. Villalobos A. Dealing with chemotherapy extravasations: a new technique. J Am Anim Hosp Assoc 2006;42(4):321–5.

102. Chamouni P, Lenain P, Buchonnet G, et al. Difficulties in the management of an incomplete form of refractory thrombotic thrombocytopenic purpura, the usefulness of vincristine. Transfus Sci 2000;23(2):101–6.

103. Ferrara F, Copia C, Annunziata M, et al. Vincristine as salvage treatment for refractory thrombotic thrombocytopenic purpura. Ann Hematol 1999;78(11): 521–3.

104. Lewis D, Meyers KM. Canine idiopathic thrombocytopenia purpura. J Vet Intern Med 1996;10:207–18.

105. Mackin AJ, Allen DG, Johnston IB. Effects of vincristine and prednisone on platelet numbers and function in clinically normal dogs. Am J Vet Res 1995; 56(1):100–8.

106. Grau-Bassas ER, Kociba GJ, Couto CG. Vincristine impairs platelet aggregation in dogs with lymphoma. J Vet Intern Med 2000;14(1):81–5.

107. Kazatchkine MD, Kaveri SV. Immunomodulation of autoimmune and inflammatory diseases with intravenous immune globulin. N Engl J Med 2001;345(10): 747–55.

108. Emmi L, Chiarini F. The role of intravenous immunoglobulin therapy in autoimmune and inflammatory disorders. Neurol Sci 2002;23(Suppl 1):S1–8.

109. Knezevic-Maramica I, Kruskall MS. Intravenous immune globulins: an update for clinicians. Transfusion 2003;43(10):1460–80.

110. Vaccaro C, Zhou J, Ober RJ, et al. Engineering the Fc region of immunoglobulin G to modulate in vivo antibody levels. Nat Biotechnol 2005;23(10):1283–8.

111. Kroez M, Kanzy EJ, Gronski P, et al. Hypotension with intravenous immunoglobulin therapy: importance of pH and dimer formation. Biologicals 2003;31(4): 277–86.

112. Marie I, Maurey G, Herve F, et al. Intravenous immunoglobulin-associated arterial and venous thrombosis; report of a series and review of the literature. Br J Dermatol 2006;155(4):714–21.

113. Cayco AV, Perazella MA, Hayslett JP. Renal insufficiency after intravenous immune globulin therapy: a report of two cases and an analysis of the literature. J Am Soc Nephrol 1997;8(11):1788–94.

114. Sekul EA, Cupler EJ, Dalakas MC. Aseptic meningitis associated with high-dose intravenous immunoglobulin therapy: frequency and risk factors. Ann Intern Med 1994;121(4):259–62.

115. Orbach H, Katz U, Sherer Y, et al. Intravenous immunoglobulin: adverse effects and safe administration. Clin Rev Allergy Immunol 2005;29(3):173–84.

116. Byrne KP, Giger U. Use of human immunoglobulin for treatment of severe erythema multiforme in a cat. J Am Vet Med Assoc 2002;220(2):197–201, 183–94.

117. Grozdanic S, Harper M, Kecova H. Antibody-mediated retinopathies in canine patients: mechanism, diagnosis, and treatment modalities. Vet Clin North Am Small Anim Pract 2008;38(2):361–87.

118. Rahilly LJ, Keating JH, O'Toole TE. The use of intravenous human immunoglobulin in treatment of severe pemphigus foliaceus in a dog. J Vet Intern Med 2006; 20(6):1483–6.

119. Scott-Moncrieff JC, Reagan WJ, Snyder PW, et al. Intravenous administration of human immune globulin in dogs with immune-mediated hemolytic anemia. J Am Vet Med Assoc 1997;210(11):1623–7.

120. Trotman TK, Phillips H, Fordyce H, et al. Treatment of severe adverse cutaneous drug reactions with human intravenous immunoglobulin in two dogs. J Am Anim Hosp Assoc 2006;42(4):312–20.

121. Bianco D, Armstrong PJ, Washabau RJ. Treatment of severe immune-mediated thrombocytopenia with human IV immunoglobulin in 5 dogs. J Vet Intern Med 2007;21(4):694–9.

122. Bianco D, Armstrong PJ, Washabau RJ. A prospective, randomized, double-blinded, placebo-controlled study of human intravenous immunoglobulin for the acute management of presumptive primary immune-mediated thrombocytopenia in dogs. J Vet Intern Med 2009;23(5):1071–8.

123. Tsuchiya R, Akutsu Y, Ikegami A, et al. Prothrombotic and inflammatory effects of intravenous administration of human immunoglobulin G in dogs. J Vet Intern Med 2009;23(6):1164–9.

124. Whelan MF, O'Toole TE, Chan DL, et al. Use of human immunoglobulin in addition to glucocorticoids for the initial treatment of dogs with immune-mediated hemolytic anemia. J Vet Emerg Crit Care (San Antonio) 2009;19(2):158–64.

125. Nuttall TJ, Malham T. Successful intravenous human immunoglobulin treatment of drug-induced Stevens-Johnson syndrome in a dog. J Small Anim Pract 2004; 45(7):357–61.

126. Ahmed AR, Dahl MV. Consensus statement on the use of intravenous immunoglobulin therapy in the treatment of autoimmune mucocutaneous blistering diseases. Arch Dermatol 2003;139(8):1051–9.

127. Chen C, Danekas LH, Ratko TA, et al. A multicenter drug use surveillance of intravenous immunoglobulin utilization in US academic health centers. Ann Pharmacother 2000;34(3):295–9.

128. Darabi K, Abdel-Wahab O, Dzik WH. Current usage of intravenous immune globulin and the rationale behind it: the Massachusetts General Hospital data and a review of the literature. Transfusion 2006;46(5):741–53.

129. Durandy A. Immunoglobulin class switch recombination: study through human natural mutants. Philos Trans R Soc Lond B Biol Sci 2009;364(1517): 577–82.

130. Foster CS, Chang PY, Ahmed AR. Combination of rituximab and intravenous immunoglobulin for recalcitrant ocular cicatricial pemphigoid: a preliminary report. Ophthalmology 2010;117(5):861–9.

131. Reagan WJ, Scott-Moncrieff C, Christian J, et al. Effects of human intravenous immunoglobulin on canine monocytes and lymphocytes. Am J Vet Res 1998; 59(12):1568–74.

132. Scott-Moncrieff JC, Reagan WJ. Human intravenous immunoglobulin therapy. Semin Vet Med Surg (Small Anim) 1997;12(3):178–85.

133. Kellerman DL, Bruyette DS. Intravenous human immunoglobulin for the treatment of immune-mediated hemolytic anemia in 13 dogs. J Vet Intern Med 1997;11(6):327–32.

134. Spurlock NK, Prittie JE. A review of current indications, adverse effects, and administration recommendations for intravenous immunoglobulin. J Vet Emerg Crit Care (San Antonio) 2011;21(5):471–83.

135. Czaja AJ. Diagnosis, pathogenesis, and treatment of autoimmune hepatitis after liver transplantation. Dig Dis Sci 2012;57(9):2248–66.

136. Danovitch GM. Mycophenolate mofetil: a decade of clinical experience. Transplantation 2005;80(Suppl 2):S272–4.

137. Ritter ML, Pirofski L. Mycophenolate mofetil: effects on cellular immune subsets, infectious complications, and antimicrobial activity. Transpl Infect Dis 2009; 11(4):290–7.

138. Drosos AA. Newer immunosuppressive drugs: their potential role in rheumatoid arthritis therapy. Drugs 2002;62(6):891–907.

139. Juel VC, Massey JM. Myasthenia gravis. Orphanet J Rare Dis 2007;2:44.

140. Orvis AK, Wesson SK, Breza TS Jr, et al. Mycophenolate mofetil in dermatology. J Am Acad Dermatol 2009;60(2):183–99 [quiz: 200–2].

141. Mehling A, Grabbe S, Voskort M, et al. Mycophenolate mofetil impairs the maturation and function of murine dendritic cells. J Immunol 2000;165(5): 2374–81.

142. Morath C, Zeier M. Review of the antiproliferative properties of mycophenolate mofetil in non-immune cells. Int J Clin Pharmacol Ther 2003;41(10):465–9.

143. Behrend M. Adverse gastrointestinal effects of mycophenolate mofetil: aetiology, incidence and management. Drug Saf 2001;24(9):645–63.

144. Chanda SM, Sellin JH, Torres CM, et al. Comparative gastrointestinal effects of mycophenolate mofetil capsules and enteric-coated tablets of sodium-mycophenolic acid in beagle dogs. Transplant Proc 2002;34(8):3387–92.

145. Dewey CW, Cerda-Gonzalez S, Fletcher DJ, et al. Mycophenolate mofetil treatment in dogs with serologically diagnosed acquired myasthenia gravis: 27 cases (1999-2008). J Am Vet Med Assoc 2010;236(6):664–8.

146. Dewey CW, Booth DM. Pharmacokinetics of single-dose oral and intravenous mycophenolate mofetil adminstraton in normal dogs [abstract]. J Vet Intern Med 2001;15:304.

147. Naderer OJ, Dupuis RE, Heinzen EL, et al. The influence of norfloxacin and metronidazole on the disposition of mycophenolate mofetil. J Clin Pharmacol 2005;45(2):219–26.

148. Gabardi S, Olyaei A. Evaluation of potential interactions between mycophenolic acid derivatives and proton pump inhibitors. Ann Pharmacother 2012;46(7–8): 1054–64.

149. Manitpisitkul W, McCann E, Lee S, et al. Drug interactions in transplant patients: what everyone should know. Curr Opin Nephrol Hypertens 2009;18(5): 404–11.

150. Lam S, Partovi N, Ting LS, et al. Corticosteroid interactions with cyclosporine, tacrolimus, mycophenolate, and sirolimus: fact or fiction? Ann Pharmacother 2008;42(7):1037–47.

151. Yuki M, Sugimoto N, Otsuka H, et al. Recovery of a dog from aplastic anaemia after treatment with mycophenolate mofetil. Aust Vet J 2007;85(12):495–7.

152. Ginel PJ, Blanco B, Lucena R, et al. Steroid-sparing effect of mycophenolate mofetil in the treatment of a subepidermal blistering autoimmune disease in a dog. J S Afr Vet Assoc 2010;81(4):253–7.

153. Bacek LM, Macintire DK. Treatment of primary immune-mediated hemolytic anemia with mycophenolate mofetil in two cats. J Vet Emerg Crit Care (San Antonio) 2011;21(1):45–9.

154. Langman LJ, Shapiro AM, Lakey JR, et al. Pharmacodynamic assessment of mycophenolic acid-induced immunosuppression by measurement of inosine monophosphate dehydrogenase activity in a canine model. Transplantation 1996;61(1):87–92.

155. Lupu M, McCune JS, Kuhr CS, et al. Pharmacokinetics of oral mycophenolate mofetil in dog: bioavailability studies and the impact of antibiotic therapy. Biol Blood Marrow Transplant 2006;12(12):1352–4.

156. Marder W, McCune WJ. Advances in immunosuppressive therapy. Semin Respir Crit Care Med 2007;28(4):398–417.

157. Pinto P, Dougados M. Leflunomide in clinical practice. Acta Reumatol Port 2006; 31(3):215–24.

158. Tallantyre E, Evangelou N, Constantinescu CS. Spotlight on teriflunomide. Int MS J 2008;15(2):62–8.

159. Gregory CR, Silva HT, Patz JD, et al. Comparative effects of malononitriloamide analogs of leflunomide on whole blood lymphocyte stimulation in humans, rhesus macaques, cats, dogs, and rats. Transplant Proc 1998;30(4):1047–8.

160. Kyles AE, Gregory CR, Craigmill AL. Comparison of the in vitro antiproliferative effects of five immunosuppressive drugs on lymphocytes in whole blood from cats. Am J Vet Res 2000;61(8):906–9.

161. Colopy SA, Baker TA, Muir P. Efficacy of leflunomide for treatment of immune-mediated polyarthritis in dogs: 14 cases (2006-2008). J Am Vet Med Assoc 2010;236(3):312–8.

162. Gregory CR, Stewart A, Sturges B, et al. Leflunomide effectively treats naturally occurring immune-mediated and inflammatory diseases of dogs that are unresponsive to conventional therapy. Transplant Proc 1998;30(8):4143–8.

163. McChesney LP, Xiao F, Sankary HN, et al. An evaluation of leflunomide in the canine renal transplantation model. Transplantation 1994;57(12):1717–22.

164. Affolter VK, Moore PF. Canine cutaneous and systemic histiocytosis: reactive histiocytosis of dermal dendritic cells. Am J Dermatopathol 2000;22:40–8.

165. Hanna FY. Disease modifying treatment for feline rheumatoid arthritis. Vet Comp Orthop Traumatol 2005;18(2):94–9.

Nutraceuticals for Canine Liver Disease: Assessing the Evidence

Jean-Michel Vandeweerd, PhD[a],*, Carole Cambier, PhD[b],
Pascal Gustin, PhD[b]

KEYWORDS

- Nutraceuticals • Dietary supplement • Liver • Evidence

KEY POINTS

- Until greater regulatory oversight of nutritional supplements is required, veterinarians will need to weigh the costs, risks, and potential benefits of nutritional supplements for their patients on an individual basis.
- Veterinarians should strive to maintain a critical view of nonscientific promotional material and rely primarily on scientific evidence.
- Before recommending or administering a nutritional supplement to canine patients with the intent of providing hepatoprotection, veterinarians should obtain informed consent from the owners to ensure they understand that little to no evidence exists to support the use of these products for the treatment or prevention of liver disease.
- Veterinarians also must be aware that lack of adequate regulation of so-called nutraceuticals increases the risk of lack of quality control, labeling inaccuracies, and omission of cautionary statements.
- Although some dietary supplements have shown beneficial effects under limited in vitro conditions or for a very specific hepatotoxin, their general use as global hepatoprotectants remains questionable.

INTRODUCTION

Therapeutic agents, called *hepatoprotectants*, have been promoted for their potential role in the ancillary treatment of liver disease in dogs and cats.[1,2] These products include both prescription drugs and nondrug dietary supplements.

A drug, by definition, refers to "any substance, food, or nonfood that is used to treat, cure, mitigate, or prevent a disease and any nonfood substance that is intended to affect the structure or function of man or animals."[3] To become a drug, a compound

Disclosures: The authors have nothing to disclose.
[a] Integrated Veterinary Research Unit (IVRU) - Namur Research Institute for Life Sciences (NARILIS), Department of Veterinary Medicine, University of Namur, rue de Bruxelles, 61, Namur 5000, Belgium; [b] Unit of Pharmacology, Department of Functional Sciences, Faculty of Veterinary Medicine, University of Liège, Boulevard de Colonster, B41, Liège 4000, Belgium
* Corresponding author.
E-mail address: jean-michel.vandeweerd@fundp.ac.be

must undergo an extensive drug approval by competent authorities such as the US Food and Drug Administration (FDA) and European Medicines Agency, and be shown to be safe and effective for its intended use.

Under the Dietary Supplement Health and Education Act of 1994, the term *dietary supplement* is defined as a product taken by mouth that contains a dietary ingredient intended to supplement the diet. The dietary ingredients in these products can include vitamins, minerals, herbs or other botanicals, amino acids, and substances such as enzymes, organ tissues, and metabolites. Dietary supplements can also be extracts or concentrates, and can be found in many forms such as tablets, capsules, softgels, gelcaps, liquids, or powders. These different definitions apply to human consumers and not pets.

The term *nutraceutical* was coined from "nutrition" and "pharmaceutical" in 1989 and was defined as, "a food (or part of a food) that provides medical or health benefits, including the prevention and/or treatment of a disease."[4] According to the North American Veterinary Nutraceutical Council, a nutraceutical is "a substance produced in purified or extracted form which, when administered orally to patients, aims to provide them the necessary elements for their structure and normal function to better their health and well-being."[3] However, the term *nutraceutical* as commonly used in marketing has no regulatory definition,[5] because only a registered drug may have indications against diseases. Because the term *nutraceutical* has no regulatory or legal definition, the authors will refer to these compounds as *nutritional* or *dietary supplements*.

For a limited number of compounds, veterinarians may find formulations that are classified as drugs if the compound is formulated one way (ie, injectable) for a specific indication, and the same or similar compounds have been classified as a nutritional supplement if formulated a different way (ie, oral) without a specific indication. The veterinarian should be assured that if the product is an FDA-approved drug, it has undergone safety and efficacy testing for the specific indication on the label. The same is not true for the nutritional supplement. One example is chondroitin sulfate, a compound frequently touted for treating canine osteoarthritis. An injectable form of polysulfated glycosaminoglycans, containing primarily chondroitin sulfate, is FDA-approved for intramuscular injection to control signs associated with noninfectious degenerative and/or traumatic arthritis of canine synovial joints. Numerous nutritional supplements containing chondroitin sulfate for oral administration are marketed, but none have undergone the rigid safety and efficacy studies required for FDA approval. Because oral bioavailability of many nutritional supplements is limited, evidence of a compound's efficacy via parenteral administration should not be used to justify its use via oral administration.

The veterinary profession has ethical obligations to ensure effective and safe treatment and to base therapeutic decisions on scientific evidence. It important to know the true efficacy and safety of products, such as dietary supplements, that are used in veterinary medicine. Because these products are often promoted as "natural," pet owners may have the misconception that they are safer than drugs. These products may be used widely by pet owners because they can purchase them directly at health food stores or on the Internet. Therefore, veterinarians must have a thorough understanding of the safety and efficacy of dietary supplements in veterinary patients. This article focuses on several dietary supplements suggested to be useful for treating liver diseases in dogs.

HEPATOACTIVE DIETARY SUPPLEMENTS: WHAT CAN BE FOUND IN THE SCIENTIFIC LITERATURE?

With MEDLINE, no "MeSH term" (Medical Subject Headings term) can be identified for "Nutraceuticals." Instead "Dietary Supplements" is proposed. When the equation

("Dietary Supplements"[MeSH] AND "Liver Diseases"[MeSH] AND "Dogs"[MeSH]) is used in MEDLINE, CAB Abstracts, and Google Scholar, very few research papers are identified. Only 9 research papers are useful for analysis (**Table 1**).[6–14] No relevant reference is identified in the databases about efficacy of vitamin E. However, very detailed narrative reviews about hepatoprotectants were published by Center in 2004 (a review of 105 pages)[2] and Webster and Cooper in 2009[15] in *Veterinary Clinics of North America: Small Animal Practice*, which provide a thorough description of the physiopathology of liver diseases (mechanisms of hepatocyte cell death, oxidative stress) and possible actions of food and nonfood products that are called *hepatoprotectants*. Dietary supplements that are commonly listed as "hepatoprotectants" include SAMe, yutan (which contains ursodeoxycholic acid [UDCA]), and silymarin (derived from the milk thistle plant).

SAME

SAMe has been marketed for use in dogs with liver disorders. It is purported to have antiinflammatory and antioxidant effects, and to play a role in cellular replication and protein synthesis. SAMe is an endogenous molecule produced from the amino acid methionine and plays a central role in the transsulfuration process that generates glutathione. Glutathione, an antioxidant and free radical scavenger, serves as a major physiologic defense mechanism against oxidative stress in hepatocytes.[2] Decreases in hepatic glutathione levels have been described in dogs and cats with severe liver disease.[13] Although specific indications for nutritional supplements are not allowed by the FDA, SAMe is often recommended as an adjunct treatment of necroinflammatory, metabolic, and cholestatic hepatopathies in dogs and cats.[15] At the recommended dose of 20 mg/kg/d orally, a low incidence of side effects has been reported.[2] Nausea or refusal of food, vomiting, and anxiety may occur in the postpill interval (hours).

Data supporting the use of SAMe in canine and feline patients is minimal. In 2002, SAMe was reported to be useful in a case of acetaminophen toxicity.[8] However, because this was a single case report, any potential beneficial effects of SAMe cannot be confirmed. In 2005, Center and colleagues[16] assessed the influence of orally administered SAMe on clinicopathologic and hepatic effects induced by long-term (84 days) administration of prednisolone in dogs. The study compared 2 groups of 4 animals (n = 8). Despite the fact that SAMe-treated dogs were not protected from the classic clinicopathologic and histopathologic features (vacuolar hepatopathy) associated with so-called steroid hepatopathy, the authors concluded that administration of 20 mg/kg/d of SAMe may mitigate the apparent pro-oxidant influences of prednisolone. Despite the lack of data supporting the use of SAMe as a hepatoprotectant, the compound is frequently recommended for dogs with hepatobiliary disease. Before veterinarians recommend use of SAMe, they should ensure that owners understand (informed consent) that data on its efficacy are lacking.

YUTAN

Yutan, a Chinese compound derived from the dried bile of the Chinese black bear, has been used for centuries for its purported hepatobiliary healing powers.[15] In 1936, UDCA was identified as the major bile acid responsible for Yutan's hepatoprotective effects.[17,18] Currently, synthetic forms of UDCA are available as an FDA-approved human drug that is specifically indicated for the treatment of primary biliary cirrhosis. Its beneficial effects may be from replacement of more toxic bile acids in the bile acid pool, stimulation of choleresis, antiapoptotic effects, stabilization of mitochondrial function, and/or immunomodulatory actions.[15] Despite its limited indication in humans,

Table 1
Articles assessing the clinical efficacy of potential hepatoprotective nutritional supplements in dogs

Title	Authors	Date	Journal	Study Design
Use of ursodeoxycholic acids in a dog with chronic hepatitis: effects on serum hepatic tests and endogenous bile acid composition	Meyer DJ, et al[6]	1997	J Vet Intern Med	Single case report
Nonsurgical resolution of gallbladder mucocele in two dogs	Walter R, et al[7]	2008	J Am Vet Med Assoc	Case report
S-adenosyl-L-methionine (SAMe) for the treatment of acetaminophen toxicity in a dog	Wallace K, et al[8]	2002	J Am Anim Hosp Assoc	Single case report
Protection by silibinin against Amanita phalloides intoxication in beagles	Vogel G, et al[9]	1984	Toxicol Appl Pharmacol	Experimental in vivo trial (induced hepatotoxicosis)
Verification of the hepatoprotective and therapeutic effect of silymarin in experimental liver injury with tetrachloromethane in dogs	Paulova J, et al[10]	1990	Vet Med (Praha)	Experimental in vivo trial (induced hepatotoxicosis)
Improvement of portal flow and hepatic microcirculatory tissue flow with N-acetylcysteine in dogs with obstructive jaundice produced by bile duct ligation	Kigawa G, et al[11]	2000	Eur J Surg	Experimental in vivo trial (induced hepatopathy)
Short-term effects of N-acetylcysteine and ischemic preconditioning in a canine model of hepatic ischemia-reperfusion injury	Baumann J, et al[12]	2008	Eur Surg Res	Experimental in vivo trial (induced hepatopathy)
Evaluation of the influence of S-adenosylmethionine on systemic and hepatic effects of prednisolone in dogs	Center SA, et al[13]	2005	Am J Vet Res	Experimental in vivo trial (induced hepatopathy)

(continued on next page)

Table 1 (continued)				
Title	**Authors**	**Date**	**Journal**	**Study Design**
Prospective randomized clinical trial assessing the efficacy of Denamarin for prevention of CCNU-induced hepatopathy in tumor-bearing dogs	Skorupski KA, et al[14]	2011	J Vet Intern Med	Experimental in vivo trial (hepatopathy associated with the use of CCNU)

Abbreviation: CCNU, Chloroethylcyclohexylnitrosourea.

it has been recommended (10–15 mg/kg/d orally) for the treatment of cholestatic, necroinflammatory, metabolic, and immune-mediated hepatopathies in dogs.[15] Three case reports represent the only scientific data supporting the use of UDCA for treating hepatobiliary diseases in the dog.[6,7]

SILYMARIN

Silymarin is derived from the milk thistle plant (*Silybum marianum*) which grows world-wide and has been used in Europe for more than 2000 years as a home remedy for liver disease in man.[19,20] A standard milk thistle extract contains 60% to 70% silymarin, which is composed of a mixture of flavonolignans, such as silibinin (silybin), isosilibinin (isosilybin), silidianin (silydianin), and silichristin (silychristin), with silibinin being the major active component.[20] Silymarin is thought to exert antioxidant, anti-inflammatory, and antifibrotic effects.[15,19] At suggested doses (50–250 mg/kg orally, twice per day),[21] no adverse effects have been reported. However, silymarin may inhibit the activity of drug-metabolizing enzymes.[15] However, silibinin has poor oral bioavailability.[22]

In 1984, Vogel and colleagues[9] investigated the use of intravenous silibinin for the treatment of amanita mushroom toxicity in beagles. A single oral dose of the lyophilized death cap fungus *Amanita phalloides* was administered to experimental dogs (n = 23). Twelve dogs served as controls, whereas the remaining 11 were treated with 50 mg/kg of silibinin intravenously at 5 and 24 hours after intoxication. The investigators subjectively reported that gastrointestinal signs were of lesser severity in animals treated with silibinin, but no objective data or scoring system was provided. Of the 12 dogs given *A phalloides* but not treated with silibinin, 4 died with signs of hepatic coma and histopathologic evidence of widespread hemorrhagic hepatic necrosis. All 11 silibinin-treated dogs survived. Although several parameters that indicate liver disease were measured (alanine aminotransferase [ALT], aspartate aminotransferase [AST], alkaline phosphatase [AP], bilirubin, and prothrombin time) neither means, medians, nor individual animal values were reported. Figures plotting these values over time were provided and the authors reported that abnormal values were less pronounced in silibinin-treated animals than in the controls. However, no statistical comparisons were made. Furthermore, it should be noted that silibinin was administered intravenously and therefore, by definition, cannot be considered a nutraceutical.

In 1990, Paulova and colleagues[10] tested the efficacy of silymarin for treating tetrachloromethane-induced liver disease in dogs. The information provided is taken from the abstract only because an English language version of the article was not available. Sixteen beagles (n = 16) were divided into 4 groups of 4 animals. Three groups were administered a dose of tetrachloromethane in sunflower oil by mouth. A negative control group was given sunflower oil only. Silymarin was evaluated separately as a preventive (silymarin administered 4 days before tetrachloromethane; n = 4) and as a treatment (silymarin administered 4 days after tetrachloromethane; n = 4). The authors reported that the ability of silymarin to protect the liver was low.

COMBINATION OF SAME AND SILYMARIN

A recent prospective randomized controlled trial assessed a commercially available veterinary product containing a stable salt of SAMe and silybin in a phosphatidylcholine complex.[14] Increased liver enzyme activity occurs commonly in dogs receiving Chloroethylcyclohexylnitrosourea (CCNU) chemotherapy (a nitrosourea alkylating agent used in veterinary medicine to treat a variety of canine cancers). Although most dogs do not develop hepatopathy to the degree that medical intervention is necessary, CCNU treatment may be delayed or discontinued to prevent potential liver failure. In this study, 50 dogs were prospectively randomized to receive either concurrent SAMe and silybin during CCNU chemotherapy (n = 25) or to receive only CCNU (n = 25). Serum biochemical profiles for hepatic parameters (ALT, AST, AP, bilirubin, and cholesterol) were analyzed before each dose of CCNU. Increased ALT activity occurred in 84% of dogs receiving CCNU alone (21 dogs) and in 68% of dogs on concurrent SAMe and silybin (17 dogs). Dogs receiving CCNU alone had significantly greater increases in ALT ($P = .03$), aspartate aminotransferase ($P = .01$), alkaline phosphatase ($P = .009$), and bilirubin ($P = .02$), and a significantly greater decrease in serum cholesterol concentrations ($P = .02$) than dogs receiving concurrent SAMe and silybin. Dogs receiving CCNU alone were significantly more likely to have treatment delayed or discontinued because of increased ALT activity. The authors suggested that SAMe and silybin can minimize the effects of CCNU on both hepatocellular damage and biliary dysfunction. The authors also objectively reported several weaknesses of their study: (1) the low number of cases that underwent additional liver testing with bile acids, abdominal ultrasound examination, and liver biopsies; (2) the low incidence of severe liver disease that may have affected results comparing changes between groups in blood urea nitrogen, albumin, cholesterol, and glucose levels, which are measures of liver function that change only when the organ is severely affected; (3) the lack of placebo in the control group, and lack of blinding of clinician as to which group each dog was assigned; (4) the occult preexisting liver disease in some dogs enrolled into the study, which may have affected results; and (5) the combination of 2 agents in the compound that was studied instead of individual products. The authors also had potential financial conflicts of interest.

VITAMIN E

Eight isomers (vitamers) of vitamin E exist, the most biologically active of which is α-tocopherol.[20] Vitamin E is synthesized by plants and is found primarily in vegetable oils, nuts, seeds, and grains. Its primary physiologic role is as an antioxidant.[15] Vitamin E is a lipid-soluble component of cell membranes that inhibits lipid peroxidation and modulates intracellular signaling pathways that rely on reactive oxygen intermediates. A dose of 15 IU/kg/d orally of α-tocopherol acetate has been recommended for dogs.[15] No adverse effects have been reported although vitamin E may inhibit the absorption of other fat-soluble vitamins when administered at high doses. In veterinary medicine, vitamin E supplements have been recommended for dermatologic and hepatobiliary diseases (cholestatic and necroinflammatory hepatopathies) in which antioxidant activity may be of benefit.[15,20] However, no scientific data support their use for any of these indications.

N-ACETYLCYSTEINE

N-acetylcysteine (NAC) is a formulation of the amino acid L-cysteine that is an FDA-approved drug for specific indications in humans, specifically as a mucolytic agent (inhalation) and acetaminophen antidote (oral). NAC is also marketed as a nutritional supplement that may have hepatoprotective effects. NAC may be used to replenish intracellular cysteine and glutathione levels, which are important for overall hepatic health.[15] Several other potentially hepatoprotective effects have been reported, including an effect on vascular tone that may improve oxygen delivery in acute liver failure, effects on hepatic mitochondrial energy metabolism, and potential effects on inflammation.[23]

A study in which obstructive jaundice was produced by ligation of the common bile duct for 7 days in 2 groups of male beagle dogs (n = 14; receiving either 5% dextrose or NAC) suggested that NAC increased the concentrations of plasma cyclic 3′,5′-guanosine monophosphate (cGMP) (intracellular cGMP elicits vasorelaxant mechanisms and plasma cGMP concentrations may be related to hemodynamic alterations in patients with cirrhosis) serum and hepatic-reduced glutathione, and hepatic adenosine triphosphate (ATP) (reduced hepatic ATP may demonstrate impaired energy homeostasis) in cholestatic-induced hepatopathy.[11] In an in vivo canine liver model of ischemic reperfusion injury (n = 15), Baumann and colleagues[12] evaluated NAC's potential protective effects (150 mg/kg injected intravenously before induction of ischemia) as determined by indocyanine green plasma disappearance rate. Plasma clearance of indocyanine green and serum levels of AST and ALT showed no significant differences between NAC-treated and untreated groups.

HEPATOACTIVE NUTRACEUTICALS: WHAT CAN BE GLEANED FROM AVAILABLE SCIENTIFIC LITERATURE?

Currently, limited available evidence exists regarding the efficacy of nutritional supplements. Two reviews detail the use of dietary supplements as hepatoprotectants for dogs,[2,15] but only 8 clinically relevant publications were referenced. Only under very limited circumstances were some nutritional supplements shown to have a favorable biochemical or clinical outcome in treating or preventing hepatic disease.

Minimal regulatory oversight of veterinary nutritional supplements may explain this lack of scientific evidence regarding the clinical efficacy of these products.[24] Because the FDA does not consider nutritional supplements to be drugs, manufacturers are not currently required to provide efficacy data as long as the label does not make medicinal claims.

When evaluating the scientific literature available for nutritional supplements, one must consider the route of administration and composition of the compound used in the research population compared with the composition of the marketed product. In some research publications, a highly purified compound with verified potency was used rather than the commercially available nutritional supplement. Additionally, using multiple nutritional supplements makes it difficult to ascertain which particular compound may have provided a beneficial effect.

SUMMARY

Until greater regulatory oversight of nutritional supplements is required, veterinarians will have to weigh the costs, risks, and potential benefits of nutritional supplements for their patients on an individual basis. Veterinarians should strive to maintain a critical view of nonscientific promotional material and rely primarily on scientific evidence. Before recommending or administering a nutritional supplement to canine patients with the intent of providing hepatoprotection, veterinarians should obtain informed consent from owners to ensure that they understand that little to no evidence exists to support the use of these products for treatment or prevention of liver disease. Veterinarians must also be aware that lack of adequate regulation of so-called nutraceuticals increases the risk of lack of quality control, labeling inaccuracies, and omission of cautionary statements. Although some dietary supplements have shown beneficial effects under limited in vitro conditions or for a very specific hepatotoxin, their general use as global hepatoprotectants remains questionable.

REFERENCES

1. Johnson SE. Chronic hepatic disorders. In: Ettinger SJ, Feldman EC, editors. Textbook of veterinary internal medicine, vol. 2, 5th edition. Philadelphia: Saunders; 2000. p. 1298–325.
2. Center SA. Metabolic, antioxidant, nutraceutical, probiotic, and herbal therapies relating to the management of hepatobiliary disorders. Vet Clin North Am Small Anim Pract 2004;34:67–172.
3. Boothe DM. Nutraceuticals in veterinary medicine, Part 1: definitions and regulations. Compend Contin Educ Pract Vet 1997;19:1248–55.
4. Brower V. Nutraceuticals: poised for a healthy slice of the healthcare market? Nat Biotechnol 1998;16:728–31.
5. Zeisel SH. Regulation of "nutraceuticals." Science 1999;285:185–6.
6. Meyer DJ, Thompson MB, Senior DF. Use of ursodeoxycholic acids in a dog with chronic hepatitis: effects on serum hepatic tests and endogenous bile acid composition. J Vet Intern Med 1997;11:195–7.
7. Walter R, Dunn ME, d'Anjou MA, et al. Nonsurgical resolution of gallbladder mucocele in two dogs. J Am Vet Med Assoc 2008;232(11):1688–93.
8. Wallace K, Center SA, Hickford F, et al. S-adenosyl-L-methionine (SAMe) for the treatment of acetaminophen toxicity in a dog. J Am Anim Hosp Assoc 2002;38: 246–54.
9. Vogel G, Tuchweber B, Trost W, et al. Protection by silibinin against Amanita phalloides intoxication in beagles. Toxicol Appl Pharmacol 1984;73:355–62.
10. Paulova J, Dvorak M, Kolouch F, et al. Verification of the hepatoprotective and therapeutic effect of silymarin in experimental liver injury with tetrachloromethane in dogs. Vet Med (Praha) 1990;35:629–35.
11. Kigawa G, Nakano H, Kumada K, et al. Improvement of portal flow and hepatic microcirculatory tissue flow with N-acetylcysteine in dogs with obstructive jaundice produced by bile duct ligation. Eur J Surg 2000;166:77–84.
12. Baumann J, Ghosh S, Szakmany T, et al. Short-term effects of N-acetylcysteine and ischemic preconditioning in a canine model of hepatic ischemia-reperfusion injury. Eur Surg Res 2008;41:226–30.
13. Center SA, Warner KL, Erb HN. Liver glutathione concentrations in dogs and cats with naturally occurring liver disease. Am J Vet Res 2002;63:1187–97.
14. Skorupski KA, Hammond GM, Irish AM, et al. Prospective randomized clinical trial assessing the efficacy of Denamarin for prevention of CCNU-induced hepatopathy in tumor-bearing dogs. J Vet Intern Med 2011;25:838–45.
15. Webster CR, Cooper J. Therapeutic use of cytoprotective agents in canine and feline hepatobiliary disease. Vet Clin North Am Small Anim Pract 2009;39(3): 631–52.

16. Center SA, Warner KL, McCabe J, et al. Evaluation of the influence of S-adenosyl-methionine on systemic and hepatic effects of prednisolone in dogs. Am J Vet Res 2005;66:330–41.
17. Beuers U. Drug insight: mechanisms and sites of action of ursodeoxycholic acid in cholestasis. Nat Clin Pract Gastroenterol Hepatol 2006;3:318–28.
18. Paumgartner G. Medical treatment of cholestatic liver diseases: from pathobiology to pharmacological targets. World J Gastroenterol 2006;12:4445–51.
19. Flora K, Hahn M, Rosen H, et al. Milk thistle (Silybum marianum) for the therapy of liver disease. Am J Gastroenterol 1998;93:139–43.
20. Flatland B. Botanicals, vitamins, and minerals and the liver: therapeutic applications and potential toxicities. Comp Cont Educ 2003;25:514–24.
21. Twedt DC. A review of traditional and not so traditional therapies for liver disease. In: Proceedings, 19th Annual American College of Veterinary Internal Medicine Forum. Denver (CO): American College of Veterinary Internal Medicine; 2001. p. 610–2.
22. Sun N, Zhang X, Lu Y, et al. In vitro evaluation and pharmacokinetics in dogs of solid dispersion pellets containing Silybum marianum extract prepared by fluid-bed coating. Planta Med 2008;74:126–32.
23. Zafarullah M, Li WQ, Sylvester J, et al. Molecular mechanisms of N-acetylcysteine actions. Cell Mol Life Sci 2003;60:6–20.
24. Vandeweerd JM, Coisnon C, Clegg P, et al. Systematic review of efficacy of nutraceuticals to alleviate clinical signs of osteoarthritis. J Vet Intern Med 2012; 26:448–56.

Index

Note: Page numbers of article titles are in **boldface** type.

Vet Clin Small Anim 43 (2013) 1181–1191
http://dx.doi.org/10.1016/S0195-5616(13)00145-9
0195-5616/13/$ – see front matter © 2013 Elsevier Inc. All rights reserved.

vetsmall.theclinics.com

Moving?

Make sure your subscription moves with you!

To notify us of your new address, find your **Clinics Account Number** (located on your mailing label above your name), and contact customer service at:

Email: journalscustomerservice-usa@elsevier.com

800-654-2452 (subscribers in the U.S. & Canada)
314-447-8871 (subscribers outside of the U.S. & Canada)

Fax number: 314-447-8029

Elsevier Health Sciences Division
Subscription Customer Service
3251 Riverport Lane
Maryland Heights, MO 63043

*To ensure uninterrupted delivery of your subscription, please notify us at least 4 weeks in advance of move.

Printed and bound by CPI Group (UK) Ltd, Croydon, CR0 4YY

03/10/2024

01040493-0018